A Whole Foods Primer

*A Comprehensive, Instructive,
and Enlightening Guide to
the World of Whole Foods*

BEATRICE TRUM HUNTER

Basic Health
PUBLICATIONS, INC.

The information contained in this book is based upon the research and personal and professional experiences of the author. It is not intended as a substitute for consulting with your physician or other healthcare provider. Any attempt to diagnose and treat an illness should be done under the direction of a healthcare professional.

The publisher does not advocate the use of any particular healthcare protocol but believes the information in this book should be available to the public. The publisher and author are not responsible for any adverse effects or consequences resulting from the use of the suggestions, preparations, or procedures discussed in this book. Should the reader have any questions concerning the appropriateness of any procedures or preparation mentioned, the author and the publisher strongly suggest consulting a professional healthcare advisor.

Basic Health Publications, Inc.
28812 Top of the World Drive
Laguna Beach, CA 92651
949-715-7327 • www.basichealthpub.com

Library of Congress Cataloging-in-Publication Data
Hunter, Beatrice Trum.
    A whole foods primer : a comprehensive, instructive, and enlightening guide to the world of whole foods / Beatrice Trum Hunter.
        p. cm.
    Includes bibliographical references and index.
    ISBN-13: 978-1-59120-086-4
    ISBN-10: 1-59120-086-5
    1. Natural foods. I. Title.

    TX369.H84   2006
    641.3'02—dc22
                                                            2006007775

Editor: Cheryl Hirsch
Typesetting/Book design: Gary A. Rosenberg
Cover design: Mike Stromberg

Printed in the United States of America

10   9   8   7   6   5   4   3   2   1

Contents

Introduction: A "Whole Food" Defined, 1

1. A Cornucopia of Vegetables, 3

2. Succulent Fruits, 37

3. Wholesome Whole Grains, 67

4. Nutrient-Dense Nuts and Seeds, 93

5. Quality Counts with Protein Foods, 119

Conclusion: Moving Forward with a Whole Foods Diet, 163

Selected References, 165

Index, 179

About the Author, 188

Dedicated to
Thomas S. Cowan, M.D.,
with homage.

A "Whole Food" Defined

Whole foods are recognized readily: cabbage, celery, carrot, and potato; apple, orange, strawberry, and watermelon; brown rice, barley, whole wheat berry, and rye berry; almond, pecan, pistachio, and walnut; sunflower seed, sesame seed, pumpkin seed, and flaxseed; egg, chicken, trout, yogurt, cheddar cheese, liver, lamb roast, beef steak, and pork chop. These are examples of foods that have been familiar to humans throughout the centuries.

Frequently, a "whole food" has been described as a food to which "nothing has been added, and nothing has been taken away." The concept is clear: "Nothing has been added" assures that the common practice of using chemical additives, such as preservatives, texturizers, stabilizers, and other substances, has not been employed. Many of these additives are used primarily to suit the technical needs of food processors; they do not necessarily benefit consumers, and some may be harmful to health. "Nothing has been taken away" assures that the common practice of refining food, resulting in a loss of nutrients, has not been employed. In any refining process, such as the conversion of whole-wheat grain into white flour, many nutrients are lost or depleted.

Yet, this definition may be simplistic. For example, a yogurt manufacturer may produce an unflavored yogurt made from organically produced whole milk, and choose to add several beneficial strains of bacteria in addition to the *Acidophilus bulgaricus* that converts the milk into yogurt. The additional strains of bacteria are unnecessary to produce the yogurt, but they provide additional benefits in the intestinal tracts of consumers. Such an addition does not fit into the definition of a whole food with nothing added.

Nor is the phrase "nothing has been taken away" always applicable. For example, if we choose to eat chicken, we may opt to eat the skin along with the flesh and organs, but surely we discard the feathers and bones. We may

1

choose to eat a roast or a steak from a steer, but we do not consume its hide or its hair. Similarly, we discard the exterior of a pineapple, the core of an apple, the skin of an avocado, and the shell of a peanut. In this sense, we are not choosing to eat a food "whole." We exclude certain parts of foods that we regard as nonedible. Perhaps a more nuanced definition of a whole food is a food that is minimally processed.

With the industrialization of food, whole foods came to be regarded merely as raw materials for further processing and refinement. Processed foods, which have longer shelf lives, were more convenient and profitable than foods in their original whole state.

The movement began in 1874, with the invention of the steel-rolling mill that replaced the stone-grinding mill for grains. The steel-rolling mill allowed for large-scale milling and speedier grinding of grain into flour. The wheat berry was partitioned. The perishable wheat germ was removed from the flour to bestow longer life to the flour. The wheat germ—the embryo of the wheat berry—could be sold profitably. The bran—the outer coat of the grain—was removed from the flour, and sold as animal feed. Other fractions were also removed and sold as byproducts. The remaining white flour—the impoverished portion of the wheat berry—did not turn rancid readily and was used in bakery products for human consumption. Partitioning the wheat berry was practical and profitable.

Later, it became far more profitable to sell potatoes as potato chips than as a whole food for boiling or baking. Similarly, it became far more profitable to sell corn as cornflakes than as a whole food of corn on the cob. Similar fractioning of food has occurred throughout all the basic food groups.

The partitioning of food has gone on apace, and stores are now flooded with partitioned food products. They are convenient, have long shelf lives, and are profitable. Unfortunately, the partitioning must be viewed as a health hazard. It lowers important nutritional offerings and destroys vital nutrient relationships. This book will demonstrate, repeatedly, the wisdom of selecting whole foods for optimal intake of nutrients that are vital to good health.

Belatedly, the importance of whole foods is gradually receiving some attention in governmental policy. The United States government's 2005 *Dietary Guidelines for Americans* made two pertinent revisions: One, Americans should increase their consumption of whole grains; and two, Americans should consume more whole fruits rather than fruit juices. These modest recommendations represent a token recognition of the values of consuming whole foods.

CHAPTER 1

A Cornucopia of Vegetables

Eat your veggies!

—SAGE ADVICE FROM EVERY CAREGIVER TO EVERY CHILD

Nutritionists tell us that it is wise to eat a wide variety of foods, every day. By doing so we have a good opportunity to obtain all the nutrients our bodies need to maintain health.

In all parts of the United States, we are blessed with a great assortment of vegetables from which to choose throughout the year. Regrettably, many Americans eat too few vegetables and limit their selection to only a few, such as white potatoes, tomatoes, and iceberg lettuce. Unfortunately, the white potato, which is consumed the most, is not apt to be eaten baked or boiled, but rather in less desirable forms as French fries and potato chips.

BEYOND NUTRIENTS: PHYTOCHEMICALS

For many years, nutritional researchers were in pursuit of basic nutrients in foods, including vegetables. They identified proteins, fats, carbohydrates, vitamins, minerals, and trace minerals. They *assumed* that they had discovered all that needed to be known to achieve an optimal diet. However, they began to find and identify other substances in foods that, like nutrients, could exert profound beneficial effects on health. These substances were phytochemicals (sometimes called phytonutrients). The name "phytochemical" is derived from *phyto*, the Greek word for plant, and is defined as a chemical that is synthesized from plants.

Identifying and understanding phytochemicals is an ongoing project. As more information is gathered, it becomes clearer that eating a variety of whole foods offers many health benefits, not only from nutrients, but from phytochemicals, too. Vegetables are especially rich sources of phytochemicals.

Remember the official 5-A-Day campaign promoted by the U.S. Department of Agriculture (USDA), encouraging Americans to eat five servings of vegetables and fruits daily? Yet many Americans still fail to meet this modest goal, despite the fact that the National Cancer Institute *doubled* the recommended number of fruit and vegetable servings to ten a day, because of newer, overwhelming findings about the benefits of these foods. Even the meager intake most Americans accomplish is apt to be made from choices that are not especially dense in nutrients or phytochemicals.

During evolution, plants developed the ability to synthesize certain chemicals to help them maintain their growth, as well as to protect them against threats such as damage from sunlight, insects, and diseases. In turn, animals that eat the plants benefit from many of the phytochemicals produced by the plants. The animals are able to maintain their own growth and protect themselves from damage, thanks to the phytochemicals in the plant food.

Certain food phytochemicals have no nutritional value but exert buffering actions, at one or more stages of cancer development. These inhibitory effects of phytochemicals on carcinogenic processes have been demonstrated in several animal models and in some experimental cell-culture studies. Numerous short- and long-term animal studies strongly suggest that certain food phytochemicals can retard cancer development markedly at different stages of its progression. Because of these findings, it is reasonable to believe that such food phytochemicals might slow down human cancer development. Numerous epidemiological studies (studies of disease in populations) strengthen the idea. These studies suggest that frequent and ample consumption of fresh vegetables and fruits is associated with lower cancer incidence, compared to infrequent and low consumption of these foods.

Many phytochemicals in vegetables and fruits have been identified as active inhibitors of carcinogenesis (cancer production). In several animal models, various phytochemicals have demonstrated their ability to retard one or more steps in the carcinogenic process. Certain phytochemicals can inactivate mutagens (substances that can induce changes in cells) and carcinogens directly; prevent formation of carcinogens; increase detoxification of carcinogens, as well as toxic chemicals and their secretions; scavenge and quench destructive, active oxygen radicals; reduce certain damage to DNA and cellular membranes; and retard cancer proliferation and cancer's promotion process. (See "The Top-Scoring Vegetables for Antioxidants" on page 6.)

Among the classes of phytochemicals that have been found to possess biological activity and can block various stages of carcinogenesis are phenolic compounds, including flavonoids. Flavonoids are commonly found in vegetables such as broccoli, cabbage, cucumber, squash, tomato, and eggplant, as well as in berries and citrus fruits.

Other plant phenolic compounds include curcumin, found in turmeric and mustard; carnosol, in rosemary leaves; and polyphenolic catechins, in berries, red wine, and tea. Most of these phenolic compounds share several biological and chemical properties with vitamins C and E: They scavenge destructive, active oxygen radicals and chemical electrophiles (electron-attracting atoms or agents). They inhibit carcinogenic formation from compounds such as nitrosamines (found in certain food products, as well as in the stomach). And they have the capacity to modulate certain cellular enzyme activities.

Sulfur-containing phytochemicals stimulate the production of detoxification enzymes and exert buffering effects against toxic chemicals, mutagens, and carcinogens. For example, allyl sulfide, a sulfur-containing phytochemical, is present in bulb vegetables, such as garlic, onion, leek, shallot, and in chive. Isothiocyanates, another sulfur-containing phytochemical group, are found in broccoli, cabbage, watercress, garden cress, and radish. Sulforaphane is in broccoli.

Indoles can modulate estrogen metabolism by degrading estrogen to forms that are less active or inactive in their ability to promote breast cancer growth. Indoles are present in cruciferous vegetables, such as broccoli, cabbage, Brussels sprouts, and cauliflower.

Carotenoids have potent antioxidant activity. Several retard cancer-cell growth. Carotenoids include vitamin A precursors and are found extensively in orange-colored vegetables and fruits, such as carrots, sweet potato, winter squash, and cantaloupe.

As more research is being conducted, it has been discovered that all vegetables are not equal in their phytochemical content. For example, Elizabeth Jeffrey, Ph.D., a nutritional scientist, and her colleagues at the University of Illinois in Urbana-Champaign analyzed fifty varieties of broccoli to measure their antioxidant and cancer-fighting compounds. The results were startling. Some varieties had as much as ten times the vitamin E content as others; eight times the beta-carotene content as others; and twice the vitamin C content as others. Also, the broccoli varieties ranged in their amounts of glucosinolates, which are phytochemicals that promote the breakdown of carcinogens and suppress cancerous tumor growth.

Another finding came from the research of Yasuko Okamoto and

Takayuki Shibamoto at the University of California at Davis and published in the *Journal of Agricultural and Food Chemistry* in 2004. The researchers discovered that a water extract of fresh asparagus totally degraded malathion within four hours. Malathion is an organophosphate pesticide commonly used over large areas for pest-eradication programs. For example, malathion has been sprayed over extensive regions to control mosquitoes that may carry West Nile virus.

Okamoto and Shibamoto noted that it is not possible to eliminate all pesticide residues from foods. Thus, their finding is an important breakthrough. Compounds exist in foods that are capable of degrading toxic pesticides. In the tests, asparagus was the best performer for this task. Next were carrots, which degraded about three-fourths of the malathion. Kale and spinach degraded some of the pesticide, but less efficiently. Broccoli degraded the least amount.

Thus, vegetables contain not only nutrients but also phytochemicals that amplify the benefits derived from these foods. Without the present knowledge of phytochemicals, the traditional advice of caregivers to children to "eat your veggies!" was even wiser than they realized—and should be heeded by persons of all ages. Eat your veggies, eat more of them, and eat a greater variety of them!

THE TOP-SCORING VEGETABLES FOR ANTIOXIDANTS

The antioxidant properties of a food are measured by oxygen radical absorbancy capacity (ORAC). This system measures a food's ability to quench oxygen-derived free radicals by comparing its absorption of peroxyl or hydroxyl radicals, common types of free radicals, to that of a water-soluble vitamin E analog. Based on ORAC, the following vegetables have the highest antioxidant properties.

Vegetable (per 100 grams)	ORAC units
Kale	1,770
Spinach	1,260
Brussels sprouts	980
Broccoli flowers	890
Beets	840
Bell peppers, red	710
Onions	450
Corn	400
Eggplant	390

Source: USDA Jean Mayer Human Nutrition Research Center on Aging at Tufts University, Boston, MA, 2000.

BUYING AND STORING VEGETABLES

Fresh vegetables usually are at their best quality and price at the peak of their season, when their supply is plentiful. But don't buy them merely because their prices are low. Buy only as many vegetables as you can use, without waste. Most fresh vegetables can be stored in the refrigerator for a few days. Root vegetables can be stored for weeks, or even months.

Whenever possible, select produce, as well as other whole foods, that are organically or biodynamically grown. Because no toxic insecticides or herbicides are used in their production, organic and biodynamic foods are better for your health.

Remember that after vegetables have been picked, they begin to lose their value in two different ways. The first loss is the obvious physical one, such as with deteriorated outer leaves of lettuce. Once harvested, they wilt. The second loss is more subtle and develops with changes in the structure of the plant tissue. Because aspiration and enzyme activity continue in harvested plants, the texture and vitamin contents of some vegetables deteriorate rapidly. This is especially true of vegetables stored improperly, at inappropriate temperatures. Visible signs are wilted or limp vegetables, or ones that have become dry, brown, or pale.

Some vegetables need to be stored with some humidity; others do best in dry air. Some do best stored in sun or in light; others need to be shielded from light. By learning the ideal storage conditions for different vegetables, you can minimize their nutritional losses.

Leafy Green Vegetables: Kale, Spinach, Chard, and Others

Refrigerate fresh vegetables such as salad greens, kale, spinach, turnip greens, and chard as soon as you bring them into the house. These vegetables retain nutrients best when stored in high humidity, at near freezing temperature. Use a vegetable crisper section of the refrigerator. Wash greens just before preparing them.

Dark-green leafy vegetables, as well as broccoli, will retain only about half of their total ascorbic acid (vitamin C) after five days in the refrigerator with the temperature between 40°F and 50°F. Even with such a substantial loss of ascorbic acid, these vegetables are still an excellent source of this vitamin (and vitamin A, as well as other nutrients and beneficial substances) due to their high initial supplies of it. Even after such loss, they may provide more ascorbic acid (and vitamin A) than freshly harvested snap beans, head lettuce (such as Bibb, Boston, and romaine), or tomatoes.

In tests to determine nutrient losses, ascorbic acid is often evaluated. This vitamin is heat, light, and time sensitive. Because of ascorbic acid's instability, it is reasoned that if this vitamin is severely depleted from a food, other nutrient losses have also occurred.

Cruciferous Vegetables: Cabbage, Broccoli, Cauliflower, and Others

Cabbage—with its many varieties—is a more stable source of ascorbic acid than most leafy green vegetables, so plan to use the more perishable ones first, and store the cabbage for later use. Even when kept at room temperature (between 65°F and 80°F), unlike most vegetables, cabbage was found to hold its ascorbic acid well. Also when kept in cold storage, under 40°F, but above freezing, cabbage retained its ascorbic acid for at least two months. However, store the cabbage in humidity, by wrapping it in a damp towel and placing it in the vegetable crisper of the refrigerator. Brussels sprouts, cauliflower, broccoli, and other members of the cruciferous family also store well in this manner.

Root and Tuberous Vegetables: Carrots and Potatoes

Carrots, white and sweet potatoes, and other root vegetables and tubers will retain their most important nutrients reasonably well if you store them in a cool place, with enough humidity to prevent them from withering. They spoil quickly if they are in direct contact with water, so do not allow condensation to form on them. If you live in the suburbs or the country, keep root and tuberous vegetables in a root cellar, a well-ventilated cool basement, an unheated pantry, or a garage. If you are an urban dweller, buy such vegetables in small quantities, and if you need to store them at room temperatures, store them only briefly.

Potatoes, parsnips, turnips, sweet potatoes, and yams are not considered exceptionally good sources of ascorbic acid, but they do contribute fair amounts of this vitamin to the daily diet. Ascorbic acid is highest in white potatoes when they are freshly dug. Immature potatoes contain more ascorbic acid than potatoes left in the ground to mature. Stored potatoes suffer a progressive loss of ascorbic acid, occurring most rapidly during the early weeks of storage. After about three months of storage, potatoes retain approximately half their original ascorbic acid supply; after six months, only one-third.

If you store white potatoes for long periods at temperatures a few degrees above freezing, they may develop an undesirable sweet flavor. However, such chilling does not harm their nutrient content. The bland flavor of the potatoes can be restored if you place them at room temperature for a few days. However, do not freeze potatoes. They will develop off-color and off-flavor features, which cannot be reversed.

Always store white potatoes in the dark. If you buy them in brown bags that contain air holes, these bags make good storage containers for the potatoes at home. If you store potatoes in light, they develop poisonous green skins. Discard such potatoes, or at least, remove all of the green portions. Never eat potato sprouts; they are poisonous. Discard blighted (diseased) potatoes. Naturally occurring chemicals, or possibly some compounds not yet identified but suspected of being toxic, may be present in blighted potatoes. They may be hazardous to health.

Sweet potatoes, like white potatoes, lose a great amount of ascorbic acid during the early months of storage, followed by a more gradual loss. At the end of three months—at which time three-fourths of the sweet potato crop has probably reached consumers—some 30 to 40 percent of the original ascorbic acid content may be lost; in six months, another 10 percent. However, retention of the sweet potato's carotene is different. After harvest, the carotene content of sweet potatoes is high. But, unlike most vegetables, their carotene content usually *increases* during the storage period before they reach retail markets. After about six months, the carotene content begins to decline. However, sweet potatoes generally are not stored longer than six months.

Cucurbits: Squash, Pumpkin, and Zucchini

Summer squashes and their diminutives consist of numerous varieties of zucca and zucchini (Italian); calabaza and calabacita (Spanish); and courge and courgette (French). These cucurbits are relatively small in size, have tender skins and flesh, and are mild in flavor. Because of their high moisture content, they are highly perishable. They do not store well. Use them promptly.

For medium-size summer squash of any variety, shred, salt, drain, and sauté or steam quickly in order to retain a crisp texture and fresh flavor. Season to taste. Winter squashes and pumpkins are available year-round. They are at their prime from fall until late winter.

Select squashes and pumpkins that are firm. Squashes that have soft spots are either immature or overmature. The stems should be full and firm. If the stems are skimpy or green, the vegetables are immature. Select pumpkins with stems intact. Once the stems are removed, the openings that remain permit bacterial entry.

The skin of these vegetables should be relatively dull, not shiny. Avoid those that have been waxed.

Recognize mature coloring of these vegetables. Pumpkins should have no green tinge if the skin color ranges from cream, to tan, yellow, orange, or red. Squash may show a lighter-colored area where the vegetables have rested on the earth. But this area should be yellow or orange, not greenish.

Select squash and pumpkin with vivid colors around harvest time, from late summer to fall. Later, during storage, the coloring may not remain so vivid, but the vegetables will be sweeter and richer in flavor.

If large squash varieties, such as calabaza, banana, or Hubbard, are too much for your needs, consider buying smaller amounts, packaged in chunks. Look for flesh that is closely grained, not fibrous. It should look barely moist, not watery or dried out.

Winter squashes and pumpkins can be kept for months, if stored properly. With long storage, these cucurbits may even improve in flavor. Store them in a well-ventilated cool area, preferably between 55°F and 60°F. It has been common practice in New England to store cucurbits under beds in unheated rooms! However, once cucurbits are cut open, they should be refrigerated.

Winter squash and pumpkin can be used as cooked vegetables. Peel and remove the seeds. Cut into chunks and simmer in a small amount of water. Season to taste. Or, after cooking, purée the chunks. Also, they can be baked or made into squash or pumpkin pies.

Bulb Vegetables: Garlic, Onion, Leek, and Shallot

Worldwide, more than 300 varieties of garlic are grown. This bulb, commonly available in the United States, is one with papery white skin and a strong flavor. It is grown mainly in California, Louisiana, and Texas. The slightly less pungent purple-skinned garlic may be imported from Mexico or Italy.

The two main varieties of garlic are softneck and hardneck. Softneck garlic is stalkless and produces many small "cloves" per bulb. The flavor ranges from very mild to very hot. Hardneck garlic produces a woody flower stalk and has large cloves. The flavor of hardneck garlic is more complex and subtle.

Select firm garlic bulbs and store them in an open container in a cool, dark place. Once a bulb is opened, the individual cloves will keep for three to ten days.

The amount of flavor released from fresh garlic depends on its preparation. The smaller the cutting, the stronger the taste, because it releases more essential oils. As a rule of thumb, the following preparations bring out the various flavors in freshly cut garlic from greatest to least strength: pressed, crushed, minced, chopped, sliced, sautéed, or baked. By cutting or pressing the garlic cloves, the garlic's cells are ruptured. This action releases an enzyme that changes its allinin content into allicin (a sulfur-containing molecule) that releases its pungent odor. Soon, the allicin decomposes into several compounds, including methyl allyl and diallyl, disulfides (also in cabbage flavor); propenyl disulfides (also in onion odor); and propenyl sulphenic acid (the compound responsible for making the eyes water).

Use garlic raw, as in salads. Or, add it to cooked vegetables, soups, or stews. The whole bulb, when baked slowly, becomes milder and sweeter than when it is raw.

Although I have tried many suggestions for avoiding eye tearing when handling raw garlic (and raw onions), none work for me. I simply accept a temporary discomfort and balance it against the increased pleasure of eating foods flavored with these pungent bulbs.

Onions, like garlic, come in many varieties. Those such as vidalia, Spanish, and Bermuda onions are mild tasting, while others such as Western Yellow and New York Bold onions are pungent. Although all onions are nutritious, the pungent ones contain higher levels of flavonoids and phenolics. According to Rui Hai Liu, associate professor of Food Science at Cornell University in Ithaca, New York, onions are the richest source of flavonoids in the human diet. Flavonoid consumption has been associated with a reduced risk of cancer, heart disease, and diabetes.

Liu and his associates conducted test-tube experiments with cancer cells from the liver and colon. They exposed the cells to extracts from different varieties of onions and shallots to learn which ones were the most effective against cancer cells. Those that were the most pungent demonstrated the greatest potential against cancer. (*Journal of Agricultural and Food Chemistry,* 2004; 52: 6787)

When shopping for onions, look for bulbs that are firm and dry. They should not show signs of mold, softness, or other indications of deterioration. Reject bulbs that have sprouted; they are past their prime. The outer paper-dry skin should be bright and smooth. Check the neck or stem end of the bulbs for signs of dampness or woody centers.

Store onions in a cool, dark, and dry area. Do not store them in proximity to stored potatoes. Because potatoes give off moisture, they may cause neighboring onions to sprout or rot prematurely.

Fresh green onions (also known as scallions) should display bright, fresh-looking tops and medium-length, clean white root ends. Store them in the refrigerator, and use them promptly. Usually, raw green onions are cut and added to a tossed green salad. Also, they can be used in soups and stews.

Leek is one of the mildest members of the onion family. Leek is available year-round, but the peak months are September to November, and once again in May.

Look for well-shaped, medium-sized leeks. The tops should be green and appear fresh. The root ends should have several inches of white skin. Avoid leeks that have obvious signs of deterioration, such as ragged or wilted greens. Overmature bulbs may split; such leeks will be tough and stringy.

Refrigerated leeks store well for a week or more. Before using leeks, wash them well. Be careful to clean out any grit that tends to collect in the neck area. An easy method of cleaning is to cut one vertical and one horizontal slit, as a cross, down the neck of a leek. Then rinse thoroughly.

You can eat cooked leek on its own: boil or braise, and season to taste. Also, leek is a good addition to soups and stews.

The shallot is a very delicately flavored bulb vegetable. In appearance, the shallot is half onion and half garlic. Its reddish brown skin has the appearance of an onion, but the bulb is divided into garlic-like cloves. The shallot's flavor also is divided between onion and garlic, but is more subtle than either of them.

Shallots are at their best when fresh, from late July to late October. After that period, they are still available, but they are ones that have been taken out of storage.

Select shallots that have bulbs about three-fourths of an inch in diameter. The outer skins should be smooth and dry and not shriveled. Reject any that are sprouting.

Keep shallots cool and dry by storing them in a tightly closed bag or jar in the refrigerator. Use them within a week or two. Minced shallots are a good addition to soups and stews.

"Fruit Vegetables": Avocado and Tomato

Is the avocado a fruit or a vegetable? Commonly, it is added to a tossed vegetable salad or puréed and spiced and made into guacamole for use as a side dish to the meal. Yet, it is also known as "alligator pear," which might favor it as a fruit. Perhaps its ambiguous classification has been resolved by its present description as a "fruit vegetable," meaning that the avocado is compatible with both fruits and vegetables.

There are numerous avocado varieties. Basically, they fall into two categories: those grown in California (a Guatemala-Mexican hybrid) and those grown in Florida (originally from the West Indies). California avocados tend to be higher in fat and calories than the Floridian varieties, and they have a creamier texture and finer flavor.

The avocado contains a high amount of monounsaturated oil (similar to olive oil). The avocado contributes fairly high amounts of beta-carotene, B vitamins, and some minerals, notably potassium and iron. It also contains some amounts of vitamins A and E.

In addition to their nutritional content, avocados offer other benefits. The ancient Aztecs in Mexico considered the avocado to be a sexual stimulant. Consequently, it was branded as a forbidden fruit. The Aztecs may not have been far off the mark. In recent times, it has been discovered that the avocado is a mood booster.

Another recent finding is that the avocado contains several active components that reduce liver damage. A study funded by the Ministry of Education in Japan, in cooperation with Kagome (a Japanese food and beverage manufacturer), found five compounds in avocado that are potent liver protectants. Researcher Hirokazu Kawagishi, Professor of Applied Biological Chemistry at the Shizuoka University in Japan, reported the findings at the International Chemical Congress of the Pacific Basin Societies in 2000 at Honolulu, Hawaii. In his study, each of the five avocado compounds was tested in rats that had been treated intentionally with a chemical that induced liver injuries. These injuries resembled those caused by viruses, suggesting that the compounds might help in the treatment of viral hepatitis (a virally caused inflammation of the liver). In the study, twenty-two different foods were fed to a group of rats with liver damage caused by galactosamine, a liver toxin. The avocado displayed the most activity of any of the foods in its ability to slow the liver damage, reflected by changes in the levels of specific liver enzymes.

In addition to their nutrients and other possible benefits, avocados are a food that tastes good. You can enjoy avocados year-round. When you purchase an avocado, you need to decide whether you want a ripe, ready-to-eat avocado, or one that is not yet ready but can be held for later use. A ready-to-eat one will yield a softness to slight pressure. One that is not yet ready to eat will be hard to the same pressure.

Store an unripe avocado at room temperature. You can speed up the ripening process by putting the avocado in a brown paper bag, closing it tightly, and storing it at room temperature. This practice confines the gases given off by the avocado that help the ripening process.

Either an uncut, ready-to-eat avocado or one that you have ripened at room temperature will keep in good condition in the refrigerator for several days. To preserve the color in a cut avocado, coat the surface with lemon juice or vinegar. Both will add a slight acidity to the avocado, which serves well if the avocado is used in salad or guacamole. If you want to keep the flavor neutral, coat the surface with milk, oil, or butter. Cover the cut surface with foil or wrap before you return it to the refrigerator for further storage.

Tomatoes are classified as a fruit, and the old terms for them, such as "love apple" or "golden apple" would seem to identify them as fruit. Yet, we generally associate tomatoes with vegetables, as they appear in vegetable salads or combined with other vegetables, such as onions and peppers.

The tomato is thought to have been a food contribution from the New World—first wild, and then cultivated in Mexico, and gradually in South America. By 1519, when the Spanish conquistador Hernandez Cortés reached Mexico, the tomato was already being cultivated carefully. Numerous varieties were being produced to mix with chilies in sauces and to be eaten with beans and other dishes. Gradually, the tomato was introduced into Europe and elsewhere. In the United States, the tomato was grown as an ornamental plant until the mid-nineteenth century, and only became a commercial crop in the 1880s. Ultimately, the tomato became one of the most popular foods.

The tomato appears in markets year-round, with May through August as the peak season. Many varieties are sold, ranging from diminutive "cherry" and "grape" tomatoes all the way to large "beefsteak" tomatoes. Some commercial tomatoes are picked green and allowed to ripen in transit or storage. Such tomatoes never achieve the full flavor of those that are allowed to ripen on the vine. "Cluster" tomatoes and hydroponically grown hot-house tomatoes have somewhat more flavor, but even these never achieve the flavor of tomatoes grown in a home garden, allowed to vine ripen, and plucked to be eaten while they still retain the warmth of the sun. Also, gardeners who grow tomatoes have access to varieties that never reach markets, because these tomatoes do not ship or store well due to thin skins.

In an attempt to produce more flavorsome commercial tomatoes that could be picked at a more mature stage of ripening than has been possible, Calgene, a biotechnology company, developed the Flavr Savr in the early 1990s. The company had spent eight years in research and development, at a cost of some $25 million. The company had produced a bioengineered tomato—the first of such foods. However, the project failed because the tomatoes had poor texture, and the Flavr Savr tomato scarcely reached the marketplace before it was withdrawn.

Tomatoes have long been known for their contribution of vitamins A and C. The levels of ascorbic acid in tomatoes vary considerably. Some factors that produce these variations, including region, plant variety, and farming practices, are beyond the consumer's control. The ascorbic acid in tomatoes grown outdoors and allowed to vine ripen in summer sunlight may contain twice as much ascorbic acid as wintertime greenhouse-grown tomatoes. Green tomatoes just beginning to turn color become a good source of ascorbic acid if you allow them full exposure to sunlight. Such tomatoes can develop more ascorbic acid than tomatoes from the same plant ripened under foliage. Also, there are regional variations. If you have a choice, remember that tomatoes produced on the West Coast are likely to have higher levels of ascorbic acid (and vitamin A) than tomatoes grown in the Midwest.

The interest in phytochemicals has led to the identification in tomatoes of beta-carotene, lycopene, and saponins, among others. Carotenoids were discussed at the beginning of this chapter (see page 5). Lycopene, an antioxidant in the carotenoid family, helps fight free radicals. Also, it appears to stimulate the immune system to battle cancer cells. If consumed regularly in the diet, it seems to offer protection against several types of cancer, including prostate, colon, rectal, and stomach cancers, and possibly breast and cervical cancers. Cooked tomatoes, in forms such as stewed tomatoes, tomato sauce, tomato soup, and pasteurized tomato juice, make lycopene much more available. The heat used in cooking tomatoes breaks down the cellular structure, and converts the molecular form of lycopene into one that is more readily absorbed by the body. A small amount of oil or butter added to cooked tomato products also may help increase lycopene absorption. Research at Ohio State University showed that lycopene in tomato soup is twice as likely to be absorbed by the body if full-fat milk, rather than skim milk or water, is added to the soup.

Saponins are a class of nutrient molecules comprising sugars hooked up to alkaloid, steroid, or triterpene compounds. Saponins have been identified in tomatoes. Saponins serve as natural antibiotics that help fight microbial and fungal infections, and protect the body from viruses. According to Venket Rao, a chemist at the University of Toronto in Canada, saponins help strengthen the immune system and protect against cancer.

When you are selecting tomatoes, make sure they are firm, without cracks, mold, or blemishes. The redder the tomato, the greater will be its lycopene content.

Tomatoes that have been picked before they redden fail to reach their best appearance or nutritive value if you place them on a warm windowsill or in the refrigerator. A bright red color fails to develop if the temperature rises above 85°F and remains at that temperature for long stretches of time. To redden tomatoes, store them out of sunlight but at room temperatures between 60°F and 75°F. Tomatoes ripened in the refrigerator are apt to become soft and watery, and decay readily.

If you grow tomatoes and have a bumper crop, pick ones that need to be used promptly. Whole tomatoes do not freeze well, but stewed ones do. Also, you can juice tomatoes in a blender or food processor and freeze the unstrained juice along with the pulp and seeds, for future use in soups. If you plan to can stewed tomatoes, follow the latest recommendations of the U.S. Department of Agriculture (USDA). Some newer varieties have been bred for lower acidity, and this needs to be taken into account for safe canning. If you have a food dryer, dried tomatoes do well.

Store tomatoes at room temperature, in a cool, dry area. Check them frequently and remove any that show signs of deterioration.

Other Vegetables: Pepper and Bean Varieties

Peppers, snap beans, and lima beans are vegetables that retain their ascorbic acid well, even at room temperature. Unlike cabbage and other cruciferous vegetables, they do not require high humidity in storage.

DIVERSIFY YOUR SELECTION

If you encounter unfamiliar vegetables while shopping, develop a spirit of adventure. Be willing to buy and try new ones. If you grow vegetables, try planting some that may be unfamiliar to you.

Below are a few of the less frequently used vegetables. How many are familiar to you?

Artichoke, French or Globe

The ancient wealthy Romans regarded the globe artichoke as a delicacy suitable for banquets. Later, during the Italian Renaissance, Catherine de Medici left Florence, Italy, to wed the King of France. She was accompanied by her own cooks and a supply of artichokes. This event signaled the beginning of the French "haute cuisine." The globe artichoke became such a popular vegetable in France that it was renamed the French artichoke. It was introduced into the United States by French colonists in Louisiana.

Look for compact, heavy globular buds with leaf scales that are tightly closed. If you find surface brown spots on the artichokes during the winter months, it means the buds were touched by frost, but the flavor is unharmed. The artichoke's quality is unaffected by its size. Smaller ones may be less expensive, proportionate to their size.

You may have been tempted to try artichokes but were discouraged because you do not know how to prepare them. To start, just before cooking, cut an inch off straight across the top of the buds, and pull off any loose leaves around the bottom, near the stem. Then, clip off the spiny tips of the leaves with a pair of kitchen scissors. Slip the artichokes into boiling water, using enough water to cover them. Cover the pot. Cook for about twenty minutes, turning each artichoke several times. Pierce the stem base with a fork. The artichokes should be tender. If not, cook them longer. Drain them, upside down. You can remove and discard the "chocks" (threadlike parts in the center) with a spoon. A grapefruit spoon with a serrated edge is especially helpful. Serve the artichokes hot or cold. Pull off the petals, one by one, and draw them between your front teeth to obtain only the tender base portion of the leaf. Discard the rest of the leaf. Cut the base of the artichoke into bite-size pieces for easy eating. This base is the portion that frequently is marinated and known as "artichoke heart."

Artichoke, Jerusalem

There is evidence that in prehistoric times, the Jerusalem artichoke was used by Native Americans. In 1605, the explorer Samuel de Champlain noted that this vegetable grew in areas of North America. Shortly thereafter, the plant was cultivated in France and, later, throughout Europe. The Jerusalem artichoke is unusual among root and tuber crops. Its reserve nutrient is inulin, rather than starch. Because diabetics can tolerate inulin better than starch, flour from Jerusalem artichokes has been used in dietary foods intended for diabetics.

This tuber has an odd shape. It looks somewhat like ginger root, both in shape and color. When selecting Jerusalem artichokes, choose ones that are firm and free of mold. To prepare, scrub with a brush, but do not peel. Wash thoroughly. Slice and boil them in water. Drain and add whatever flavors appeal to you, such as olive oil, garlic, and herbs. The flesh of cooked Jerusalem artichoke tends to turn oyster gray in color and tastes somewhat like water chestnut.

Cardoon

The cardoon, or cardoni, is an edible thistle, related to the globe artichoke. The cardoon has been cultivated since the days of ancient Rome and is native to the Mediterranean region. It is a good source of potassium, iron, and calcium.

This vegetable looks like large stalks of celery, with a gray-green bloom on the leaves and inner core. Choose leaf stalks that are free of blemishes and have a fresh-looking bloom. Cardoon reaches the market in fall and winter. When you are ready to use it, wash the leaf stalks and cut off the prickly edges. Remove the strings from the stalks, because these cellular strings will not soften during cooking. Boil in water. Drain and add flavorings, and serve as a cooked vegetable.

Celeriac

Celeriac, or celery root, is cultivated for its starch-storing root, rather than for its stalk. Its gnarled turniplike form, with dangling rootlets, is also known as knob celery or turnip-root celery. Celeriac is more popular in Europe than in the United States. It is a fair source of iron, calcium, and vitamin B.

This root vegetable appears in markets from October through April. Select firm, clean celeriac. Wash and scrub it with a brush to remove dirt, leaves, and rootlets. Leave the root unpeeled and whole. Cook in boiling water until tender. Then drain, peel, and slice it, and add your choice of flavorings.

Fennel

Fennel, also known as finocchio or anise, has been used since ancient times. It was cultivated by the Egyptians and also was popular with Greeks and Romans. The word "fennel" is derived from a Latin word for a kind of sweet-smelling hay that was used to repel pestiferous insects. Fennel contains some vitamin A, niacin, and some iron.

This bulb has bright green, featherlike leaves, and a mild licorice flavor. It is sold from October to March. You can use fennel as a cooked or raw vegetable. Wash and scrape any blemishes from the bulb, and prepare it as you would prepare celery. Add slices of it to a tossed salad.

Kohlrabi

Kohlrabi originated in northern Europe and was described as early as 1554. By the early 1800s, kohlrabi was being cultivated in the United States. The bulb of the vegetable contains vitamin C and the leaves, vitamin A.

This bulb vegetable appears in markets during the summer and fall, but it is at its peak of goodness in June and July, when it is harvested. Look for small- to medium-size bulbs with fresh green leaves. When the bulbs grow very large their texture becomes woody. Avoid deeply scarred or blemished bulbs. To prepare kohlrabi, pare off the skin, wash the bulb, and slice it thinly. Save the leaves if they are fresh and tender, and cook them along with the bulb. Serve as a vegetable.

Okra

Okra pods appear on the market throughout the year, but their peak months are from June through November. Select crisp, bright green pods, free of blemishes. The best okras are small to medium in size, about one to three inches in length. Wash and trim the stem ends. Leave the pods whole, but cut large ones into half-inch slices. Cook as green beans, and serve plain. Okra is an excellent soup thickener.

Rappini

Rappini (also called rapini, broccoli rabe, or broccoli raab) is a Mediterranean vegetable with a fresh Kelly green color and few buds. It appears on markets in fall and winter. Rappini is a member of the brassica family, along with broccoli, and is pungent and somewhat bitter. Remove any discolored stems, and trim the roots. Parboil, drain, and braise, boil, or steam until tender.

EATING VEGETABLES: RAW OR COOKED?

Although foods in a raw state may offer good nutrition, raw food is not for everyone. Salad greens and raw fruits should be part of a mixed diet for most people. However, the digestive tract of some people cannot tolerate large quantities of raw foods, although cooked foods may be tolerated. For anyone who has consumed mostly cooked foods for years, any radical shift to an all-raw-food diet can spell disaster.

Salad greens should be eaten raw, but many vegetables need to be cooked. Some naturally occurring toxins such as oxalic acid in spinach and rhubarb, for example, are rendered less poisonous by heat. Even the water or liquid used in cooking may serve a useful purpose by diluting the toxins. Many plant foods such as beans (legumes) and soybeans contain antinutrients, substances that can inhibit the proper absorption of nutrients. Cooking improves the digestibility of foods with antinutrients.

Cooked foods are less likely than raw foods to cause allergic reactions.

Usually, proteins are the offensive allergenic components in foods. Cooking denatures the proteins, and renders the foods less allergenic.

At-risk patients, such as those with severe burns, patients receiving cancer treatments, persons with indwelling catheters, AIDS patients, and others whose immune systems are impaired, are highly susceptible to infections. Such persons should be discouraged from eating raw foods. The most frequent infections result from the consumption of raw tomatoes, radishes, and celery. *Pseudomonas aeruginosa* and *Klebsiella* are the most troublesome contaminants affecting debilitated individuals. Some hospitals eliminate raw vegetables completely from patients' food trays. In some hospitals dealing with cancer patients, all raw food is treated with radiation to kill pathogens on food before it is served to patients. *More cancer patients die from infections than from the disease.*

However, for those who can tolerate raw foods, eating salads is one of the easiest ways to consume healthful amounts of greens and other vegetables. In this section, we will first look at shopping and preparing salads and then move on to discuss cooked vegetables.

Shopping for Salad Greens

Select greens that are fresh, crisp, and deep green. Limp greens, or those with yellowing leaves are apt to be past their prime, tough, and bitter. For the best nutritional buys, select lettuce or cabbage heads that still have lots of outer leaves; the well-trimmed heads are apt to be old. The outer leaves of lettuce, cabbage, and other greens are the ones highest in carotene; the inner leaves contain far less. For this reason, alone, the greens you purchase should be organically grown, because conventionally grown greens have the greatest amount of pesticide residue on the outer leaves.

Both the intensity of the vegetable's greenness, and the part of the plant from which it comes, are clues to its food value. Generally, the more intensely green the vegetable, the richer its content of nutrients. For example, choose dark green pascal celery rather than blanched stalks, green endive rather than Belgian endive, and Bibb lettuce rather than iceberg lettuce. Dark green leaves may carry several times as much of some nutrients as that contained in their stalks. So, plan to use the leaves of pascal celery as well as the stalks.

Expand the variety of greens you commonly choose for salads. If you have a vegetable garden, you can buy seeds for many delicious types of salad greens that rarely are grown commercially because they are too tender or perishable to ship, or they do not store well. Occasionally, you may be fortunate in finding some "native" produce sold as local surplus in a food store, or locate it at a bona fide "truck farm" roadside stand, or at a farmers' market. Types of salad greens vary in different regions of the country. Be adventurous, and try any special offerings in your area.

Following is a selection of salad greens that can be found in most places, in season.

Beet Greens

Beet greens are sometimes sold separately, especially when young beet plants are thinned out early in the growing season. Use the young, tender beet greens sparingly in salads due to their oxalate content.

Cabbage, Chinese

Chinese cabbage, sometimes called Napa or celery cabbage, is crisp with a slight anise flavor. Use Chinese cabbage like other cabbage, shredded in salad. Choose solid heads.

Cabbage, Green or White

Use the shredded leaves of green or white cabbage as a salad ingredient. The green is preferable to the white.

Cabbage, Red

This variety is interchangeable with green cabbage. Red cabbage is somewhat higher than green cabbage in some nutrients (notably magnesium).

Cabbage, Savoy

Although savoy cabbage, bright green and crinkly with a tangy mustard flavor, is usually cooked, a small amount of it is tasty in a mixed green salad.

Celery

Celery stalks and leaves should have a crisp, fresh appearance. Avoid wilted stalks or yellowed leaves.

Chicory

The lacy leaves of chicory (or curly endive) spread out, dark green on the outside and yellow at the center. The entire head of chicory, with its slightly bitter taste, mixes well with other salad greens. If the outer leaves are very large and bitter, use them as a cooked vegetable.

Dandelion Leaves

Two varieties of dandelion leaves reach the market in spring. One is cultivated, with long, pale green leaves and a mild flavor; the other is field
grown, has shorter, darker leaves, and is more bitter. Reject any dandelion
leaves if the stems already have blossoms; at this stage they are unduly bitter. Dandelion leaves, in small amounts, mix well with other salad greens.
Also, they can be cooked as a vegetable.

Endive, Belgian or French

The Belgian, or French endive is a long, narrow, very pale yellow and firm-
headed green that has tightly packed, pointed, waxy leaves. Belgian endive
has an unusually tangy flavor, and its light color forms a contrast to deeply
colored leaves in a mixed salad.

Escarole

Escarole is distinguished by its dark green, flat leaves. The outer leaves may
be bitter, in which case cook them as a vegetable. Use the less bitter inner
leaves for salad.

Fennel

As mentioned earlier, fennel (also called finocchio or anise) is a white bulb
with bright, featherlike green leaves and a mild licorice flavor. Use fennel
sparingly in a mixed salad so that the flavoring does not overpower the
other greens.

Field Salad

Field salad (also called field lettuce or lamb's tongue) is a salad green that
appears on the market infrequently. It consists of very small spears on delicate stems. At times, it is a component in mesclun, a medley of salad greens,
also known as "spring greens."

Lettuce

Several types of lettuce have been developed, including loose leaf or non-
heading lettuce (leaves that form from a stem rather than from a core); but-
terhead (with soft leaves grown in a closed head); cabbagehead (with a
closed head of crisp leaves); cos or romaine (with a tall or elongated head);
and stem lettuce or celtuce (grown for its thick stem, rather than its leaves).
Of the different types, head lettuce is most popular.

Bibb lettuce has a miniature, fragile head and is considered by many people to be the choicest of lettuce. Each leaf shades from green at the edge to yellow toward the center. It is grown in limestone soil, which is why it is sometimes called limestone lettuce. Unfortunately, Bibb lettuce is not always available, and when it is, it is often pricey.

Boston lettuce is one of the common varieties of head lettuce. It has a dark green, loosely formed head. Select a quality head of medium weight in relation to its size. If you squeeze it gently, the head should give slightly. Look for outside leaves that are fresh and green and that separate easily.

Iceberg lettuce is another common and popular variety of head lettuce. It is pale green and watery, with a compact head. It has a very bland flavor, almost insipid, is low in nutrients, and should be the least favored choice.

Leaf lettuce frequently is grown in a home garden. The leaves are soft, tender, long, fragile, and flavorsome. Alas, it neither ships well nor keeps well. Occasionally, it is found in markets. If you have your own vegetable garden, among many delicious varieties available are oak leaf, red leaf, salad bowl, Simpson, and the seldom planted one, stem lettuce.

Romaine or cos lettuce, with its long, narrow head and oval leaves, dark green outside and yellow heart, is a crisp, juicy, firm, and tasty lettuce. It stores well. Select romaine lettuce with fresh-looking crisp leaves with a minimum of blemishes. The outer leaves may be coarse, with heavy midribs. Shred such leaves for salad, or cook them as greens.

Parsley

Although most people use flat-leaf or curly leaf parsley sparingly as garnishes, both tangy varieties can be used in quantity in salads. Parsley is highly nutritious, being rich in beta-carotene, chlorophyll, iron, vitamin C, and other nutrients. Select bunches that are deep green and crisp.

Watercress

A pungent salad green, sold in bunches, watercress is identifiable by its many small, round, and dark leaves. Watercress gives a lively color to a mixed salad, as well as a zesty flavor. Select bunches with bright, deep green, crisp leaves. Prop the bunch in a glass of water, refrigerate, and use promptly.

Non-Greens in the Salad

Although greens are the primary base for a vegetable salad, many other items can be added. Among them are avocado; cucumber; onion; sweet red,

yellow, orange, and green peppers; radish; scallion; shallot; various tomatoes, including beefsteak, plum, cherry, grape, cluster, and yellow; and garlic. If herbs are not already part of your salad dressing, use them as salad
ingredients. Mince fresh chive with a pair of kitchen shears. Try, at different
times, fresh basil, chervil, dill, marjoram, mint, oregano, rosemary, sage,
savory, or thyme. Use them sparingly—a little goes a long way.

For variety, add whole, hulled sunflower, pumpkin, or sesame seeds to
salads. Nuts also make good additions. At different times, try some crushed
seeds, such as anise, caraway, celery, coriander, cumin, dill, fennel, or poppy.
Use them sparingly.

Dressing Up Your Salads

Salad dressings not only supply flavor to the greens, they also make an
important contribution to the daily diet: the oils used are a source of nutrients such as essential fatty acids (EFAs). Learn to make a basic dressing;
then, vary it as you like.

The two basic ingredients of salad dressings are oil and vinegar (or
lemon juice). Select these ingredients with care, and obtain the best quality
you can find. The customary ratio is three parts oil to one part vinegar.

Oil

Although many vegetable oils are available, the top choices are flaxseed oil
(an excellent source of EFAs) and olive oil (a predominately monounsaturated oil).

Oils should be stored in dark bottles or tins. Buy oils in small quantities,
and plan to use them promptly. Most oils are highly perishable. Once you
open the bottle or tin, close it tightly and refrigerate. Olive oil is an exception.
Once the bottle or tin is opened, close it tightly, but keep it in a cool dry place,
out of the refrigerator. It is more stable than other oils. If the bottle is clear,
store it in the dark.

Flaxseed oil is a rich source of omega-3 fatty acids (alpha-linolenic acid)
and omega-6 fatty acids (linoleic acid). Both of these fatty acids are essential
nutrients necessary in the human diet to maintain health.

On average, flaxseed oil contains 54 percent omega-3 fatty acids, 15 percent omega-6 fatty acids, and 21 percent of the nonessential but highly beneficial omega-9 fatty acids. Flaxseed oil also contains the antioxidant
nutrients beta-carotene (72 international units [IU] per tablespoon), mixed
carotenoids (1,000 micrograms [mcg] per tablespoon), and vitamin E (alpha-
tocopherol: 2.81 IU per tablespoon).

EFAs are part of the membranes of each and every cell in the body. They produce prostaglandin families, which are hormonelike substances necessary for cell-to-cell biochemical functions that are vital for various body processes such as energy metabolism, as well as for cardiovascular and immune system health. Tissues in the brain and nervous system are comprised of more than 50 percent EFAs. Yet, according to nutritional studies, the average American diet supplies only 20 percent of the required amount. Most likely, this deficiency is due to the dramatic increase in the consumption of refined vegetable oils, hydrogenated oils (used in margarine, crackers, baked goods, and in many other processed foods), and fried foods over the last few decades.

Flaxseed oil is highly perishable. It should be in a dark container. Once the container is open, close it tightly and refrigerate.

Olive oil contains relatively little alpha-linolenic fatty acids, but it has modest amounts of linoleic acids. In general, oils from plants such as the olive tree, grown in the Mediterranean region, have lesser amounts of omega-3 fatty acids than plants grown in cooler, northern regions.

Olive oil contains mostly nonessential monounsaturated fatty acids (MUFAs). Its linoleic acid (omega-6) content ranges from 3.5 to 20 percent (averaging 10 percent). Its alpha-linolenic (omega-3) content ranges from 0.1 to 6 percent. Its oleic acid (omega-9) content ranges from 63 to 83 percent (averaging 75 percent). Its palmitoleic acid (omega-7) content ranges from 0.5 to 3 percent (averaging 2 percent).

Olive oil offers numerous health benefits. Its oleic acid assists omega-3 fatty acids to enter cell membranes to help maintain the fluidity and function of cell structure. Also, oleic acid decreases the oxidation of low-density lipoproteins (LDLs), thus reducing their potential to induce atherogenesis. Also, olive oil contains palmitic acid, a saturated fatty acid. Usually palmitic acid raises cholesterol levels. However, the palmitic acid in olive oil seems to protect arteries. At present, the mechanism is not understood. Olive oil contains about 2 percent stearic acid, a neutral fatty acid that neither raises nor lowers cholesterol levels.

Olive oil contains several minor but important components, including the antioxidants beta-carotene and tocopherols (vitamin E fractions). Unrefined green olive oil contains chlorophyll, which is rich in magnesium, a mineral in short supply in many diets. Also, olive oil contains squalene, a substance that helps to deliver oxygen to tissues, especially tissues that are low in oxygen. Squalene increases heart activity, dilates blood vessels, and inhibits atherosclerosis. In addition, olive oil contains phytosterol compounds (such as beta-sitosterol) that protect against cholesterol absorption from foods. Thus, phytosterols help lower cholesterol levels. Polyphenols, plant compounds present in unrefined olive oil, have antioxidant activities that help to stabilize the oil.

Olive oil can vary considerably in quality. "Extra virgin" olive oil, which has the most distinctive flavor, is made from the first pressings of top-quality olives. In the most expensive brands, the olives are pressed in a manually operated press. Such oil is termed "pressed" or "expeller pressed," in contrast to oils that are "solvent extracted" by means of harsh chemicals. Large commercial operations use hydraulic presses to express the oil.

Disregard the term "cold pressed," which is meaningless. Only the first few drops of oil pressed out are actually cold. "Virgin olive oil" is pressed, but the olives are not always top quality. "Pure olive oil" is the lowest grade, and can be made from the second, or even third, pressing from the same olives used to make virgin olive oil.

Vinegar

In addition to oil, the other basic ingredient of salad dressings is vinegar (or lemon). Vinegar may be the byproduct of fermented beverages. Many types of vinegar are excellent for salad. Apple cider, malt, wine, and balsamic vinegars are the most familiar ones.

In recent years, balsamic vinegar (*aceto balsamico*) has become especially popular in America, due to its mellow, sweetish flavor. In centuries-old archives in Italy, balsamic vinegar was described as a tonic, a digestive, a condiment, and a liquor. The Italian word "balsamico" is thought to relate to balm—to connote a healing potion. Among Italian connoisseurs, finely aged balsamic vinegar is regarded as a fine old port wine, to be enjoyed and used sparingly. Commonly, only a few drops are used with salad greens, fruits, or other foods.

Genuine balsamic vinegar is produced in and around Modena, Italy. Unlike ordinary wine vinegar, quality balsamic vinegar is made from crushed tart Trebbiano grapes, which are allowed to ferment. As the liquid ages and evaporates, it is transferred into smaller and smaller wooden barrels. The barrels may be made from chestnut, cherry, ash, mulberry, locust, or even juniper. Each wood gives a distinctly different flavoring to the vinegar.

Balsamic vinegar is allowed to age for at least twelve years in these barrels. Yearly, the vinegar loses from 10 to 25 percent of its volume. The flavor mellows, the consistency thickens, and the amber color darkens. There is a sweet-and-sour balance. It is time-consuming and costly to produce bal-

HOMEMADE VINEGARS

Homemade vinegar is easy and inexpensive to make.

• **Apple-cider vinegar:** The simplest method for making apple-cider vinegar is to allow sweet cider to turn to vinegar. Or, if you grow apples, you can make apple-cider vinegar from apple wastes. Put the peelings, cores, and bruised apples into a thick, earthenware, wide-mouth crock. Cover the contents with cold water. Cover the crock. If the cover is not tight, place several layers of cheesecloth between the crock and the cover to keep fruit flies out. Store the crock in a warm place. From time to time, add fresh peelings, cores, and bruised apples. The "mother," a mass that forms on top of the liquid, is an active force that converts the mixture to vinegar. After several months, when the vinegar tastes strong, strain, bottle, and cork it. Save the mother as a starter to hasten fermentation in a subsequent batch, or share it with friends.

• **Malt vinegar:** To make malt vinegar, dissolve 3 pounds of hop-flavored malt extract and 2 pounds of honey in 3 quarts of hot water. Allow the mixture to cool. Then, combine it with 2 gallons of cold water. Pour the mixture into a 5-gallon crock. Soften one cake of baking yeast (or 1 tablespoon of dry-yeast granules) in $1/4$ cup of warm water. When the mixture foams, add it to the crock. Cover the crock with three layers of cheesecloth, and place the cover over the crock. Store at room temperature (70–75°F). Stir the mixture daily. On the fifth day, strain the mixture through a few layers of cheesecloth. Wash the crock thoroughly, and return the mixture to it for a second stage. Add 3 quarts of warm vinegar, which can be from a previous batch of malt vinegar, or from any other vinegar. Add a pint of raw apple juice, which you can make by juicing about $1\,1/2$ pounds of sound apples in a juicer, blender, or food processor. Strain the juice, and add it to the crock. Cover the crock and store it at room temperature for a few days. The surface will develop a film. Allow the film to remain undisturbed on top of the liquid for about a month. The mixture will develop a distinctly acidic taste. Carefully remove a sample with a spoon and taste it. When the taste has reached a desired strength, skim and strain the liquid, pour it into clean glass bottles, and cork tightly.

This recipe makes about $3\,1/2$ gallons of vinegar. It can be used immediately or allowed to ripen further in the bottles. In time, it will mellow and have a distinctive flavor. It keeps indefinitely. Save a portion of this batch to use as a starter for a subsequent one.

• **Herb vinegar:** Use any vinegar you fancy. Use either fresh or dried herbs. Basil, dill, mint, or tarragon are especially good. Fill a clear glass jar with the vinegar and the selected herb. Cover and allow the jar to stand for two weeks in a sunny window. Each day, shake the jar. When the flavor tastes sufficiently strong, strain out the herb, rebottle, and cork. Herbed vinegar makes an inexpensive but welcomed gift.

• **Wine vinegar:** Keep the unused portion of an opened bottle of dry wine, uncorked or uncapped but covered with several layers of cheesecloth, for several weeks. Gradually, the wine will convert to wine vinegar. Strain, rebottle, and cork.

• **Beet vinegar:** Beet vinegar is also called rosel or russell. It is a clear, bright red vinegar with a winelike aroma. It is used during the Jewish Passover and is an ingredient in a Russian-type beet soup. Peel and quarter a dozen large beets. Place them in a stone crock and cover them with enough cold water so that the liquid reaches to within an inch of the crock's top. Cover the crock with cheesecloth, and tilt the crock cover at a slight angle to allow some air to enter the crock. The tilting can be achieved by placing a small object, such as a stone or a piece of cutlery, between the rim of the crock and the crock's cover. Allow the mixture to stand at room temperature until it turns to vinegar, which takes about three to four weeks. Skim the surface carefully, strain, bottle, and cork.

samic vinegar, and the final product is very expensive. What most Americans purchase as balsamic vinegar is a commercial version in which wine vinegar is used as a base, and then cut with "must," the juice expressed from grapes. There is a wide range of prices for balsamic vinegar, and a wide range of quality, too. Unfortunately, the higher priced ones do not automatically guarantee that they will be superior to the lower priced ones. When you find one to your liking, note the brand for future purchases.

Other vinegars, less common, include products made from grape juice, oranges, pineapple, and honey. Vinegar does a lot to help dress up your salads. (To make your own vinegar, see the inset on pages 27–28.)

Note: Unlike apple-cider vinegar or other vinegars fermented from fruits, distilled white vinegar is made from grains, such as corn or rye. It is more pungent and used mainly as an inexpensive pickling agent. (It is useful, too, as a cleaning agent—especially when added to water, for window cleaning!) However, it is a poor selection for salad dressing.

Vegetables That Improve with Cooking

Some otherwise healthful vegetables and fruits contain toxic and undesirable substances. Spinach and rhubarb contain high levels of oxalic acid. This toxin blocks calcium absorption and can cause severe liver damage. These foods should be cooked to reduce the oxalic acid content. Cooked spinach and a calcium-rich food is a good combination. The calcium buffers the effects of the residual oxalic acid in the cooked spinach. The leaves of rhubarb should *never* be eaten, raw or cooked, because they contain high levels of this toxin. Fortunately, rhubarb's appearance in gardens and grocery stores is for a limited time in spring. It is far from ideal as a year-round food. If eaten, it should be consumed sparingly.

Red cabbage, broccoli, Brussels sprouts, cauliflower, and kale—all otherwise nutritious vegetables—contain substances called goitrogens. Goitrogens block the uptake of iodine by the thyroid gland and can lead to the development of goiter, a condition that is characterized by a swollen thyroid gland. By cooking these vegetables, the goitrogens are destroyed or greatly reduced.

In general, hard, cellulose-rich vegetables are digested better after they are cooked. The cooking process breaks down the cell walls of food and makes nutrients more readily available. Thus, vegetables such as broccoli, cauliflower, and carrot yield more nutrients when they are eaten cooked than when they are eaten raw. Cook such vegetables only long enough to loosen the fibrous matrix that encases them and locks in the nutrients. The common practice of filling appetizer platters with raw carrot sticks and cauliflower and broccoli florets, along with dips, is actually unwise.

Anyone who chooses carrots as a reliable source of vitamin A should select mature carrots and cook them. The vitamin A is locked into the fibrous matrix and is released only by cooking. Older, mature carrots contain more vitamin A than so-called baby carrots. Raw carrots should not be given to young babies, who have not yet developed the acidity present in adult stomachs. Raw carrots can ferment inside of babies' stomachs. However, babies can tolerate cooked strained carrots.

Generally, the human body has no problem absorbing vitamin C from foods. A joint study conducted by the Agricultural Research Service of the USDA and the National Cancer Institute (NCI) found that although broccoli contains vitamin C, eating it raw was about 20 percent less effective in raising vitamin C levels in human blood than other foods. It requires lots of chewing to get the maximum benefits from foods such as broccoli, when raw.

Cooking vegetables has other benefits as well. Cooking increases the palatability and digestibility of some foods. These features result in more appeal, greater consumption, and increased nutrient intake. With some phytochemicals in vegetables (see the discussion of phytochemicals at the beginning of this chapter), cooking improves their absorption. For example, lycopene, a carotenoid, protects our cell membranes from free-radical damage and DNA mutations. The tomato is a good source of lycopene, which is absorbed best when the tomato has been heat processed, as cooking releases lycopene. Products such as bottled tomato juices, tomato sauce, tomato paste, and even tomato ketchup are better sources of lycopene than raw tomatoes. Tomato sauce with olive oil, fat-containing cheeses or fat-containing ground meats, all yield appreciable amounts of lycopene. Although red-pigmented fruits such as watermelon, pink grapefruit, blood oranges, and guava are good lycopene sources, because these fruits are eaten raw, their lycopene is not as bioavailable as lycopene from cooked tomatoes.

Cooking sweet corn increases its disease-fighting antioxidants. In studies conducted at Cornell University in Ithaca, New York, Rui Hai Liu, Ph.D., and his colleagues stripped kernels from ears of fresh sweet corn and heated them at various temperatures and for different lengths of time. The researchers found that the higher the cooking temperature and the longer the heating time, the greater became the concentration of phenolic acids. Cooking released these potent and beneficial antioxidants, found in many foods, which otherwise are bound to the plant's fiber and are unavailable for absorption by the human gut. The antioxidants in the cooked corn can neutralize free radicals. Canned corn, tortillas, and some bakery products made with corn are among many food products that use heat-processed corn.

Retaining Nutrients in Cooked Vegetables

It is important to cook vegetables only long enough to loosen the fibrous matrix that surrounds the nutrients. Use as little water or other cooking liquid as possible. Use a pot with a tight-fitting lid. Steam, pressure-cook, or microwave the vegetable only until it is fairly tender; it should retain its color and still have a bit of crunch.

Stir-frying is another cooking method that works well. Because it is fast and done without water, water-soluble nutrients do not leach out. In fact, the light oil coating on the vegetables helps to retain nutrients. Also, the oil helps us to utilize the food's fat-soluble vitamins, such as vitamins A, D, E, and K. The tab of butter added to a cooked vegetable achieves the same goal. Also, it increases palatability. Beta-carotene is absorbed best in the presence of butter or oil. Thus, stir-frying carrots helps us obtain this beneficial phytochemical. Similarly, antioxidants in spinach are far better absorbed when butter or oil is added to the cooked vegetable.

In a series of tests conducted by Gertrude Armbruster, Ph.D., and her colleagues at the Department of Nutritional Sciences at Cornell University, investigators found that ascorbic acid in cooked vegetables decreased as the cooking time and amount of water was increased. In general, the lowest levels of ascorbic acid were found when vegetables were boiled. Steaming was somewhat better. For example, broccoli contained about 81 milligrams (mg) of ascorbic acid per 100 grams after boiling; 125 mg after steaming; and 162 mg after microwaving. Similar results were achieved with asparagus, Brussels sprouts, cabbage, and cauliflower.

PRESERVING VEGETABLES FOR FUTURE USE

Fresh, locally grown, picked-when-ripe-and-rushed-to-market vegetables may be best, but what happens when less-than-ideal conditions prevail? Fresh produce may be harvested in the West and shipped thousands of miles to the East. Produce selected to survive this long journey may have been picked when immature, reaching its destination in an imperfect state of ripeness. The days spent in transit inevitably cause some nutrient decline as well.

Vegetables can be preserved for future use by various means—canning, freezing, drying, root cellaring, pickling, and fermenting. Which preservation methods are best?

Freezing

Freezing preserves many nutrients in vegetables and offers a means of processing these foods at their peak of ripeness. Sweet corn and green peas are notable examples of vegetables that retain their garden-fresh qualities better when frozen than when they are "fresh" but shipped long distances.

Some vegetables are available frozen but rarely, if ever, found fresh in markets anymore. Lima beans are an example.

Some vegetables grown in the South—such as okra, which is a staple of Southern cooking—may be found in the North occasionally, frozen but rarely fresh.

If you live in a section of the country with cold winters, the supply of fresh produce reaching your market during the winter months may be quite limited. Frozen vegetables can supplement the supply of fresh ones and add greater variety to your daily diet.

If you buy commercially frozen vegetables, select plain ones without sauces. Transfer the containers promptly to your home freezer or to the freezer compartment of the refrigerator. Never thaw and then refreeze vegetables. Both their flavor and nutrients will decline.

Hold frozen vegetables well below freezing to preserve their nutrients. If you hold them merely at their freezing points, they will show a progressive loss of nutrients. Store frozen vegetables only for a limited period of time.

The recommended maximum storage period for home-frozen vegetables in a home freezer kept at 0°F is eight to twelve months. Kept at that temperature, frozen beans, broccoli, cauliflower, and spinach lose one-third to three-fourths of their ascorbic acid within a year. If you can store them as low as -20°F, such vegetables will hold far more of their ascorbic acid. Unfortunately, most home freezers are not constructed to operate at such a low temperature. If you are unable to maintain your freezer well below 0°F, plan to buy commercially frozen vegetables in small quantities and replenish the supply frequently. Date the containers before you put them in the freezer, and rotate your stock.

If you freeze homegrown vegetables, you will wish to stock a large supply in the freezer to enjoy for a long time. Although their ascorbic acid content may decline, other nutrients that are less sensitive to long storage will be retained. Minerals are an example. Follow good procedures in freezing, and blanch vegetables when recommended by the USDA or county extension service. Use airtight containers for storage.

According to experts, tomatoes do not freeze well. Yet tomatoes are usually in abundance during harvest for the home gardener. Some people do freeze tomatoes successfully by cutting them into wedges (unpeeled and raw) and placing them in containers for freezing. When thawed, these tomato wedges can be used for soups, stews, and casserole dishes.

Canning

Canning subjects vegetables to high heat and results in some nutrient losses. Some water-soluble vitamins leach into the liquid and can be retrieved if the liquid is used for soup, stew, or sauce. Commercially canned vegetables have a good record of safety. Home canning must be done carefully to prevent botulism, a severe, potentially life-threatening form of food poisoning. Newer findings show that some phytochemicals present in certain vegetables are rendered *more* available after the foods are heat processed.

Drying

Drying of vegetables can be done outdoors in the sun or indoors with a homemade or commercially purchased dehydrator or dryer. Properly dried, uncooked food has only about one-sixth to one-third the bulk of its fresh form, and only about 10 to 20 percent of the water content. However, vitamins such as ascorbic acid, which is sensitive to heat, light, and air, are reduced in the drying process. Foods dried and stored properly will last indefinitely. Any discoloration shows deterioration. Any that develop mold should be discarded.

The USDA's Cooperative State Research, Education, and Extension Service has published pamphlets on home drying. Consult your local Extension Service for the latest information. Other publications that are helpful include the following:

- *Garden Way's Guide to Food Drying* by Phyllis Hobson (Workman Publishing Co., 1983) has a good discussion of how to build an electric food dehydrator, features of commercial food dehydrators, and how to dry foods in the sun, oven, or homemade dryer.

- *Putting Food By* by Ruth Hertzberg, Beatrice Vaughan, and Janet Greene (Plume Books, 1992) contains a section on drying vegetables.

- *Keeping the Harvest* by Nancy Chioffi and Gretchen Mead (Storey Publishing, 1991) contains a chapter on drying foods, along with illustrations, photographs, and charts.

- *Solar Food Dryer* edited by Ray Wolf (Rodale Press, 1981) gives complete blueprints and instructions for building a home solar food dryer.

Root Cellaring

Root cellaring is a simple no-processing way to store vegetables, if you have the space. This system requires little work, just a free area and good storage conditions. A useful book is *Root Cellaring* by Mike and Nancy Bubel (Storey Publishing, 1991).

Pickling

Many vegetables such as cucumbers, turnips, and radishes can be pickled, and most cookbooks devote some space to this technique. Pickling bears some resemblance to canning, with a boiling water bath to help destroy bacteria, molds, yeast, and enzymes that might cause spoilage in the pickled vegetables.

Fermenting

Fermenting vegetables is among the best—if not *the very best*—method for preservation. The fermentation process involves no cooking. It depends on lactic acid and salt for fermentation. Fermentation not only retains nutrients but actually *increases* the levels of some of them. For example, ascorbic acid *increases* when cabbage is converted to sauerkraut. Fermented vegetables are readily digested, help to maintain a healthy flora in the intestinal tract, and produce antibiotics and anticarcinogens. Also, they taste good! It's no wonder fermented vegetables have long been used in traditional diets. Korean kimchi, for example, is a medley of fermented vegetables.

Although sauerkraut is a commonly recognized fermented vegetable, often it is canned and contains an excessive amount of salt. Raw sauerkraut, lacto-fermented with whey and little salt, is an entirely different product. Cabbage is only one of numerous vegetables suitable for fermentation. Others include root vegetables (daikon radish, black radish, carrot, beet, rutabaga and purple top turnip, and kohlrabi); bulb vegetables (onion and garlic); and "fruits" of vegetables (green pepper, sweet red pepper, and cucumber). Many people are acquainted with cucumber pickles made with

How to "Put By" Sauerkraut

You can make good sauerkraut from fresh cabbage year-round; just make sure the heads are sound and solid. Select green or red cabbage, or use a combination of both. For variety, try Chinese cabbage after you have mastered the process.

Remove the outer leaves, and core the cabbage. Cut away any decayed or bruised portions.

Shred the cabbage finely with a shredding device, a sharp knife, or a food processor. Put the shreds in a large mixing bowl.

Traditionally, ordinary table salt has been used for sauerkraut making, as well as for dry salting of other vegetables. My own preference is sea or earth salt, available in health/natural food stores, by mail order, or in some specialty sections of supermarkets. Among several existing brands, one is Celtic Sea Salt, which is hand harvested in Brittany, sun dried, and maintains more than eighty of its minerals. The salt is certified by Europe's Nature et Progrès, an independent third-party group, to be free from pesticides, herbicides, and other harmful chemicals. For more information about Celtic Sea Salt, or to order by mail, contact The Grain and Salt Society (273 Fairway Drive, Asheville, NC 28805; 800-867-7258; www.celtic-seasalt.com).

To make lacto-fermented sauerkraut, in addition to the shredded cabbage and salt, one more ingredient is needed: whey. If you make yogurt cheese (see "How to Make Yogurt Cheese" on page 147), you will obtain an ample amount of whey. From every quart of yogurt, you will have a pint of curd (yogurt cheese) and a pint of whey. This liquid whey will keep well for months in the refrigera-

vinegar, but not with fermented cucumbers made with whey and salt.

Sauerkraut has a venerable history. You may think of it as a traditional German dish (*sauer* meaning acid or sour, and *kraut* meaning cabbage), but actually the use of fermented cabbage probably originated in ancient China. As early as the third century B.C., this food sustained Chinese workers engaged in building the monumental Great Wall. The nomadic Central Asian Tartars carried sauerkraut westward. The ancient Romans used it as food and medicine. The Vikings, whose supply of fresh food was exhausted before the end of long voyages, wisely stored ample supplies of sauerkraut on their vessels before departure. James Lind, the noted eighteenth-century British surgeon, observed that Dutch ships carried huge barrels of *zourkool* to prevent scurvy among the sailors. This practice was long in use before the

---

tor. However, if you do not make yogurt cheese, you can buy plain powdered whey in a health/natural food store. Store it in a tightly closed jar in a cool, dark place at room temperature. Reconstitute the whey in water. If you plan to make sauerkraut on a regular basis, save the sauerkraut juice and add it to the newly made batch of sauerkraut along with the whey and salt.

Now, you have assembled the basic ingredients for sauerkraut: shredded cabbage, salt, and liquid whey. For each medium-sized head of cabbage, add 1/4 cup of liquid whey, plus a tablespoon of salt. If you wish, add a tablespoon of caraway, celery, fennel, dill, or anise seeds. The optional addition adds flavor, and these seeds are "digestives" as well, that is, they benefit digestion.

Scrub your hands and mash the ingredients together. The salt will draw out juice from the cabbage. Continue this mashing until you have produced a substantial amount of liquid. Then, pack the mixture into a clean wide-mouth glass jar, place a plate on top of the mixture, and press down until juice covers the plate and all of the sauerkraut is submerged. If one plate does not exert enough pressure, place one or two more plates on top of it within the crock, until the weight is sufficient to hold the cabbage shreds under the liquid. Cover the jar with its lid. Place the jar in a warm, dark cupboard for four days. By then, you can smell the fermentation. Remove the plates, return the jar's lid, and refrigerate. The sauerkraut is ready to be eaten.

Note: In filling the jar, allow one inch of headspace to prevent overflowing during fermentation. As an added precaution, place a tray under the jar while the cabbage is fermenting. If the jar is too large and inconvenient for storage in the refrigerator, transfer the finished sauerkraut into smaller containers. The refrigerated sauerkraut has a long shelf life.

discovery that limes and lemons were antiscorbutic (anti-scurvy) agents. Captain Cook carried thousands of pounds of cabbage on his ship to prevent the ravages of scurvy among his sailors.

Sauerkraut gives us all the valuable nutrients of cabbage, as shown by scientific investigations, and supplies them in a palatable and more easily digested form than raw or cooked cabbage. Louis Pasteur described sauerkraut as one of the most useful and healthful of all vegetable dishes.

For people who grew up in nineteenth-century rural America or Europe, making sauerkraut was a common experience. It was not unusual for a single family to process hundreds of cabbage heads for sauerkraut. This autumn activity was as regular as making pickles, jelly and jam, or drying, curing, smoking, or cellaring foods. In the nineteenth century such food-preserving activities were known as "putting by" food, and helped to feed the family during winter.

With today's supermarket offerings, you may not feel the urgency to "put by" foods. Nevertheless, there are reasons to make homemade sauerkraut. Today's commercial product is apt to be cooked, bleached with sulfur dioxide, preserved with benzoate of soda, and excessively salty. All of these negative features make the commercial product very different from homemade sauerkraut, which is uncooked, lacto-fermented, tangy and pleasant tasting, and far less salty.

Fortunately, sauerkraut is easy to make. (See "How to 'Put By' Sauerkraut" on page 34.) It requires no special ingredients, skills, or equipment. Nor do you need to prepare a hundred heads of cabbage. A single head will do! This basic method of preparing cabbage for lacto-fermentation is applicable to many other vegetables. For recipes, an especially helpful book is *Nourishing Traditions* by Sally Fallon with Mary Enig, Ph.D. (Trends Publishing, 1999).

Commercially available fermented vegetables, sometimes called "cultured" vegetables, or "lacto-fermented" vegetables, are sold at some health/natural food stores under the brand name Deep Root Organic. If you cannot find a source, you can order them by mail from Caldwell Bio-Fermentation Canada, Inc. (189, de la Rivière Road, Martinville, Quebec, JOB 2AO, Canada; 819-835-9277; www.biolacto.com). Their products are prepared from organically grown vegetables.

CHAPTER 2

Succulent Fruits

The healthiest way to eat fruit is fresh and raw,
with the skin on.

—PAUL A. LACHANCE, PH.D., PROFESSOR OF FOOD SCIENCE AND NUTRITION,
RUTGERS UNIVERSITY, FROM *FOOD PROCESSING* (JULY 2003)

Although the phrase "fruits and vegetables" seems to equate these two types of produce, they are not equal. The main emphasis should be on vegetable consumption. One can hardly overconsume broccoli, Brussels sprouts, or kale, but it is all too easy to overindulge with sweet fruits.

Unfortunately, the U.S. Department of Agriculture (USDA) groups fruits and vegetables into a single category, with the recommendation to eat at least five servings daily. As previously noted, the National Cancer Institute doubled this recommendation. Also, this advice is too vague. One could equate French fries with Swiss chard, or orange juice with blueberries. In these two examples, the foods are not equally beneficial.

Not all fruits are equal. Many Americans limit their fruit consumption to oranges, apples, and bananas. In season, they may add some grapes, strawberries, and watermelon. Many Americans are drinking fruit juices, rather than eating the fruits whole. Even worse, they often select fruit drinks that contain little real fruit juice or that are totally synthetic concoctions, consisting of sugar, fruit flavorings, coloring, and a slew of additives, but devoid of nourishment.

In the past, the USDA's Food Guide Pyramid failed to distinguish between fruit juices and whole fruits, so people wrongly assumed fruit juice to be as good as the whole fruit. It is not. One can ingest more fruit juice than one can eat whole fruits. This is undesirable. The body is assaulted by a quick surge of a high level of fruit sugar, and lacks the buffering effect of the dietary fiber that is present in the whole fruit. The fiber present in the fruit slows the rate of the fruit-sugar absorption. The 2005 revised Food Pyramid advises "moderate" use of fruit juices but fails to explain the reason.

Nonetheless, fruits are a valuable contribution to the mixed diet, provided that they are not overconsumed. Fruits are a good between-meal or road-trip snack. For snacking, choose fruits that you can wash in advance and are easy to peel, such as navel or temple oranges, tangerines, or clementines. Also, prewashed apples, pears, bananas, peaches, apricots, nectarines, grapes, and cherries are all easy to manage. Keep a knife and paper napkins in your car or at your workplace so that you can handle fruits easily.

CHAMPION FIGHTERS AGAINST FREE RADICALS

In recent years, investigators have found that, beyond vitamins, minerals, and trace minerals, fruits also contain beneficial phytochemicals. Phytochemicals, already discussed in Chapter 1, are compounds with powerful disease-fighting antioxidant properties. Among the phytochemicals found in fruits are carotenoids (beta-carotene, lutein, lycopene); flavonoids (anthocyanins, bioflavonoids, hesperidin, isoflavones, proanthocyanadins, anthocyanosides, quercetin, and rutin); phenols (polyphenols, quercetin and phloretin glycosides, chlorogenic acid, and epicatechin); ellagic acid; and resveratrol.

During normal metabolism, oxygen can form damaging byproducts called free radicals. Free radicals are molecules with an odd number of electrons. They are highly reactive and, if not quenched, can do bodily harm. The single molecules attempt to match up with other unpaired electrons. When they succeed, the next molecule (a free radical), in turn, tries to find another unpaired electron. This chain-reaction process can form thousands of free radicals quickly. In the process, cells are damaged. Scientists believe that this damage can lead to serious health problems, including heart disease, cancer, Alzheimer's and Parkinson's diseases, and even aging.

Antioxidants can bind free radicals before they cause damage. Antioxidants from foods, such as fruits, appear to have a stronger effect than antioxidants from dietary supplements. The USDA measured antioxidant levels in more than 100 foods. The agency released a list of the top twenty foods that are the best free-radical fighters, due to their antioxidant activity. Fruits, and especially berries, predominate. The list includes wild and cultivated blackberry, blueberry, cranberry, raspberry, and strawberry, as well as sweet cherry, plum and black plum, prune, and the apple varieties Red Delicious,

Granny Smith, and Gala. Other foods that made the list are some beans (small red, pinto, red kidney, and black), two cooked vegetables (artichoke and Russet potato), and among nuts, the pecan.

BERRIES: THE MOST NUTRIENT-DENSE FRUITS

Berries appear to be the most nutrient-dense fruits. Many different types of berries are available fresh during a limited season, and in frozen form year-round. Frozen berries retain their nutrients. Choose frozen berries that are plain and whole, without any added sugar or syrup. Some berries are available in dehydrated form, but these may contain added sugar. Include a variety of berries, such as blackberries, blueberries, raspberries, and strawberries, in your diet year-round.

Berries are enjoyed for their sweetness, succulence, and flavor. But there is more to savor, as an accumulating amount of scientific evidence demonstrates that berries contain potent phytochemicals that offer significant health benefits.

Among the valuable phytochemicals are the dark red berry pigments, called anthocyanins (a group of flavonoids). According to Jan Mills, president of Artemis International (a supplier of natural colors and berry extracts to food processors), anthocyanins "are powerful antioxidants with greater protective power than vitamins C and E, or beta-carotene. Anthocyanins help maintain healthy tissue and retard some of the aging processes." (*Food Product Design*, Nov 1999)

Anthocyanins have been associated with a reduced risk of heart disease. Research conducted at the University of Graz in Austria showed that the anthocyanins in standardized elderberry extract decreased oxidation of low-density lipoprotein (LDL) cholesterol, the so-called unfavorable form of cholesterol, which is implicated as a major factor in cardiovascular diseases, especially heart attack and stroke. Also, anthocyanins have been associated with reduced adhesion of platelets to blood vessel walls, which reduces the risk of atherosclerosis. Platelets are blood-cell fragments that are involved in blood clotting.

Antioxidants in blueberries, strawberries, and blackberries, as well as in sweet cherries, may fight arterial disease by preventing the oxidation of unfavorable LDL cholesterol. The oxidation of LDL is an important step in the development of heart disease. Oxidized cholesterol is thought to initiate inflammation of blood vessel walls and lead eventually to plaque buildup. This finding suggests that the phenolic compounds found in such berries may have potential cardiovascular benefits. In one experiment, researchers found that the blackberry in laboratory culture dishes displayed the greatest antioxidant activity of all fruits. Next, in descending order, were the pear, red grape, apple, cherry, strawberry, watermelon, blueberry, banana, and green grape. Although fresh fruits tested best, those that were frozen, canned, or dried still supplied ample quantities of antioxidants. The cranberry contained significantly more disease-fighting phenols than any of the other fruits tested.

The USDA's Jean Mayer Human Nutrition Research Center on Aging at Tufts University utilized standardized berry extracts to study and quantify the capacity for berry anthocyanins with the ORAC assay. The researchers found that berries rated very high in ORAC assays. (See "The Top-Scoring Fruits for Antioxidants" on page 41.) Further research, using elderberry extract, showed that anthocyanins present in the berry are well absorbed by humans. This finding is important in establishing effectiveness.

Findings from recently conducted research at Ohio State University's James Cancer Hospital and Solove Research Institute have demonstrated some health benefits from berry consumption. Rat studies showed that certain types of berries, especially black raspberry and strawberry, could reduce the incidence of esophageal and colon cancers for 60 to 80 percent of the cases. According to Gary Stoner, head of the Laboratory of Cancer Chemoprevention and Etiology at Ohio State University, similar research is being conducted throughout the country.

Jointly, researchers at the USDA's Agricultural Research Service and at Clemson University in South Carolina are investigating an assortment of berries, as well as muscadine grapes, for their ability to inhibit the growth of cell lines cultured from breast and cervical tumors. Extracts of berries, obtained using various solvents and different parts of berries, such as the juice, skin, and seeds, were utilized in tests for assays in the cancer cell lines. The findings showed that extracts from the raspberry, strawberry, and muscadine grape cut the growth of breast cancer and cervical cancer cell lines by more than half. Extracts from the blueberry and blackberry were not effective against two cervical cancer cell lines, but they did suppress breast cancer cell growth. Each type of berry suppressed different cell lines.

In rats, berries have been shown to inhibit the metabolism of some carcinogens, so that fewer mutational changes occur that can lead to cancer. Also, berries appear to slow down the growth rate of precancerous cells.

In one study reported in 1998 and led by Laura Ann Kresty at the Ohio State University College of Medicine in Columbus, researchers fed cancer-induced rats a diet of 5 to 10 percent freeze-dried black raspberries for nine

THE TOP-SCORING FRUITS FOR ANTIOXIDANTS

The antioxidant properties of a food are measured by oxygen radical absorbancy capacity (ORAC). This system measures a food's ability to quench oxygen-derived free radicals by comparing its absorption of peroxyl or hydroxyl radicals, common types of free radicals, to that of a water-soluble vitamin E analog. Based on ORAC, the following fruits have good antioxidant properties.

Fruit (per 100 grams)	ORAC Units
Prunes	5,770
Raisins	2,830
Blueberries	2,400
Blackberries	2,036
Strawberries	1,540
Raspberries	1,220
Plums	949
Oranges	750
Red grapes	739
Cherries	670
Kiwi fruit	602
Grapefruit, pink	483

Source: USDA Jean Mayer Human Nutrition Research Center on Aging at Tufts University, Boston, MA, 2000.

months. The diet reduced malignant cancer tumor development by 80 percent.

Similar to their earlier studies on esophageal cancer, also reported in 1998, a twenty-five-week study conducted in rats showed that strawberries and black raspberries reduced the esophageal cancer incidence by 50 to 60 percent. In clinical trials, to learn if these findings can be extended to humans, researchers focused on two precancerous conditions: Barrett's esophagus and familial adenomatous polyposis (FAP). In the former condition, chronic acid reflux causes the lining of the esophagus to undergo cellular changes, which lead to a type of cancer called esophageal adenocarcinoma. The latter condition, FAP, is a rare genetic disease in which colon polyps develop. If left untreated, the polyps can lead to colorectal cancer.

Can berries reduce these two precancerous conditions? Berries contain many polyphenolic compounds that have been shown to possess antimutagenic (protective against cellular mutations) and antioxidant properties. However, researchers suspect that other phytochemicals may play roles in reducing these precancerous conditions, too.

Among the phytonutrients are phenolic compounds. More than 4,000 phenols have been identified in plants. When phenol-containing plants are eaten, these compounds may protect against heart disease, certain forms of cancer, and other health problems.

The greatest phenolic content is present in the cranberry, pear, grape, apple, and blueberry, according to Joe Vinson, Ph.D., professor of chemistry at the University of Scranton in Pennsylvania. As part of his research, Vinson measured the quantity and quality of phenols. Vinson concluded that, "in terms of gram weight and serving sizes, cranberries won hands down." Vinson's findings confirmed earlier ones. He added, "Cranberries are loaded with antioxidants and should be eaten more often." Frozen and dried cranberries retain their antioxidant content. A half cup of cranberries contains 373 grams (g) of phenols; one medium pear, 317 g; a half cup of red grapes, 296 g; a medium-size apple, 256 g; a half cup of cherries, 231 g; 8 medium-size strawberries, 195 g; and one large wedge or 2 cups of diced watermelon, 183 g. (*Journal of Agricultural and Food Chemistry*, 19 Nov 2002)

Resveratrol, a potent antioxidant and anticancer agent, has been well publicized as a constituent in red wine. However, it is present as well in the blueberry, cranberry, and huckleberry. Resveratrol provides health benefits such as protection against cardiovascular diseases.

Using gas chromatography and mass spectrometric techniques, scientists from the USDA's Agricultural Research Service, in a collaborative effort with Rutgers University in New Jersey and AgCanada, an agricultural station in Kentville, Nova Scotia, measured the resveratrol content of thirty whole-fruit samples of blueberry, cranberry, huckleberry, and related berries representing five families and ten species of *Vaccinium* fruits. The samples varied in their amounts of resveratrol. Analysis of the extracts of the skin, juice, pulp, and seed of the muscadine grape showed that its concentration of resveratrol was highest in the fruit's skin. Levels in the juice and pulp were much lower than either in the skin or seeds.

In research conducted elsewhere, different species of berries were shown to vary in their content of flavonoids, ellagic acid, and polyphenolic acids. The blueberry and bilberry were rich in an antioxidant, hydroxycinnamic acid; the cranberry and lingonberry contained large amounts of flavonoids; and both the strawberry and red raspberry were high in ellagic acid.

An unanticipated discovery made by Dr. Sepp Porta, an Austrian endocrinologist, was that elderberry extract showed a capacity to reduce stress. Human subjects were given stress tests. Those who had consumed elderberry extract for ten days were tested for stress biomarkers. Measurements of glucose (blood sugar), magnesium, and other plasma chemical levels indicated that elderberry extract significantly decreased susceptibility to stress, and also shortened recovery time from physical exertion.

Gradually, researchers are discovering the identity and characteristics of phytochemicals in berries, as well as in other fruits and vegetables. The USDA, in collaboration with the Produce for Better Health Foundation, is building a database that notes specific phytochemicals that are present in individual types of fruits and vegetables.

DISTINGUISHING THE BERRIES

Shrubs of the genus *Vaccinium* produce many commonly eaten berries. The bilberry and the whortleberry, popular in Great Britain, are similar to our familiar blueberry. The cranberry is native to North America. Other relatives are the loganberry, the foxberry, and in England, the cowberry.

Among other berries is the chokeberry, which is native to the Midwest and to some Mountain States. Small and round red, white, and black currants are available widely in North America, Europe, and Asia. Black currants are popular in Europe for making tea to soothe a sore throat.

Blackberries are used in Great Britain and northern Europe for making a tea to relieve indigestion. Gooseberries are grown and eaten in France and England. Elderberries are native to Europe, Asia, and North America. Although elderberries are used in making jams, pies, and wine, they have long been used medicinally. The bark, stems, leaves, roots, and *unripe* berries contain toxins, including a bitter alkaloid and hydrocyanic acid (cyanide). The *ripe* berries are edible. They contain antioxidant activity greater than vitamin C or E. Their anthocyanins enhance immune function. They also offer cardiovascular benefits, and have antiviral activity.

There are many types of raspberries. The strawberry is a distant botanical relative of these cane berries. Loganberry is a cross between raspberry and blackberry. Boysenberry is a raspberry hybrid.

Shrubs of the genus *Morus* produce mulberries. The red mulberry is native to North America. Both black and white mulberries originated in Asia.

The following are specific characteristics of the most commonly eaten berries.

Blueberries

For centuries, blueberries have been esteemed in folklore, both as foods and as medicines. Native Americans consumed the leaves, roots, and fruits of high-bush blueberries to cure certain ailments.

In 1999, Japanese researchers demonstrated the usefulness of blueberries in improving weak eyesight and lessening eye fatigue. A follow-up survey showed that more than 85 percent of Japanese people were aware of the eyesight benefits derived from blueberry consumption.

Europeans have long consumed bilberries, a variety of blueberries, as part of their diet, especially for eye health. We have learned that a pigment in bilberries contains anthocyanins, the potent antioxidants that are thought to contribute to eye health. During World War II, pilots in the Royal Air Force ate bilberries. The pilots found that the berries helped their night vision when they conducted nighttime bombings.

Using analytical tools, including ORAC, USDA researchers developed a methodology that allowed them to measure high-antioxidant activity in anthocyanin-rich berries. At the USDA Jean Mayer Human Nutrition Research Center on Aging at Tufts University, Ronald L. Prior, Ph.D., head of the Phytochemical Laboratory, and his colleagues measured antioxidants in fruits and vegetables. They examined more than forty fruits and vegetables common in the American diet. Among berries, blueberries had the highest antioxidant capacity in the ORAC test. The bilberries from Germany scored highest. However, low-bush blueberries from Nova Scotia and other cultivars from the United States were nearly as high, depending on their stage of maturity. Naturally ripened blueberries not only taste better than berries picked before their prime but also may be more healthful than berries picked early for distant shipments.

The researchers found a threefold difference in the blueberry's ability to quench oxygen-derived free radicals, depending on the species and the maturity at harvest. Also, the researchers found that $1/2$ cup of blueberries had as much antioxidant activity as $3/4$ cup of strawberries, $1\frac{1}{2}$ cups of orange segments, $2\frac{1}{4}$ cups of broccoli florets, $2\frac{1}{2}$ cups of chopped spinach, and $2\frac{2}{3}$ cups of corn.

The wild variety of blueberries harvested commercially in Maine and eastern Canada showed the greatest amount of antioxidant activity. Those berries are smaller than cultivated ones: there are about 1,600 small, wild blueberries in a pound, compared to about 500 larger cultivated ones per pound. The flavor of the wild berries was found to be more intense, and the nutrient content of frozen wild blueberries (without added sugar) matched the nutrient content of fresh blueberries. (*Journal of Agricultural and Food Chemistry*, 1998; 46: 2686–2693)

Studies show that blueberries exert an effect similar to that of cranberries in promoting urinary tract health. In 1998, a research team at Rutgers University identified proanthocyanins, a group of phytochemicals, present in blueberries and cranberries that prevent *Escherichia coli* (*E. coli*) from adhering to the urinary tract. This bacterium leads to urinary tract infection (UTI). Thus, blueberries and cranberries showed yet another health benefit. (A discussion on cranberries follows this section.)

Another recent Tufts University project, funded jointly by the USDA and the National Institute on Aging, headed by James A. Joseph, Ph.D., chief of Tufts' neuroscience laboratory, found that aging rats fed a diet rich in blueberry extract showed markedly improved short-term memory, balance, and coordination. Lack of all these features is regarded as a key indicator of age-related decline. In the studies, the rats were given extracts of blueberry, strawberry, or spinach for eight weeks. The rats were nineteen months old— an age equivalent to a sixty-five-to-seventy-year-old human. All three extracts improved short-term memory, but only blueberry extract improved balance and coordination as well. Previous studies had linked high-antioxidant fruit and vegetable consumption to preventing dysfunction. According to Joseph, this was the first study to demonstrate a reversal in dysfunction. In the next phase of the research, clinical trials will determine whether the beneficial results with rats can be extended to humans. (*Journal of Neuroscience*, 1999; 19: 8114–8121; and Dr. Joseph's abstract "Successful Brain Aging and Polyphenolic Intake," published by the American Chemical Society, August 2002)

Investigations of blueberry's contribution to eye health have found that blueberry consumption increases circulation of the capillaries of the eyes, which reduces oxidation in these tissues. This action benefits eyesight. It is thought to be especially helpful in preventing diabetic retinopathy, as well as night blindness, macular degeneration, and cataracts.

Constituents in blueberries also are thought to strengthen all other capillaries, arteries, and veins, and to reduce capillary fragility and permeability in conditions such as varicose veins. Also, it is thought that blueberries inhibit enzymes that may promote cancer; reduce histamine production; and act as an anti-inflammatory nutrient to connective tissue.

Blueberries contain a wide range of phytochemicals, as well as beta-carotene and vitamins C and E. These components and nutrients act as antioxidants that scavenge free radicals.

In addition to blueberry, and especially bilberry, other red berries are associated with improved microcirculation and strengthening of blood vessels; viral suppression; and antioxidant, anti-inflammatory, and anticarcinogenic actions within the human body.

According to Leslie Wada, Ph.D., R.D., a nutrition consultant, "Probably the greatest immediate interest is in the antioxidant effect of berry-based anthocyanins. Consumers are becoming aware of the association between free radicals and chronic diseases such as cancer and cardiovascular ailments, and the benefits of antioxidants in helping to prevent the formation of free radicals." (*Food Product Design,* Nov 1999)

All the good news about blueberries has been hailed by the media. The University of New Hampshire's Cooperative Service bulletin heralded the blueberry as "the super food of the new millennium." The blueberry was named "Fruit of the Year" by one magazine and "the miracle berry" by another.

Cranberries

Experiments give some credence to the folk remedy of drinking cranberry juice to reduce urinary tract infections (UTIs). It has been found that certain components of cranberries interfere with the ability of *E. coli* to adhere to the cells that line the urinary tract. Chemist L. Yeap Foo and coworkers at Industrial Research, Lower Hutt, New Zealand, studied cranberry extracts and isolated three procyanidins, one of which was shown to inhibit *E. coli* from adhering to cell surfaces in laboratory tests.

Other researchers found that cranberry extract was also effective in inhibiting *Listeria monocytogenes* and *E. coli 0157:07,* two virulent foodborne pathogens. Yet, the cranberry extract allowed *Lactobacillus fermentum,* beneficial lactic acid bacteria, to thrive. This finding suggests that cranberries may affect the microbial ecology of the human gut in a positive way by inhibiting the growth of certain foodborne pathogens, yet allowing beneficial probiotic bacteria to grow and protect the gut.

Studies show that cranberries are rich in phenolic compounds, including bioflavonoids, anthocyanins, procyanidins, and phenolic acids. Some of these compounds may account for the cranberry's antibacterial activity. Also, constituents isolated from cranberry extract show antitumor activity in leukemia, and in breast, prostate, lung, and cervical cancer cell lines.

Unfortunately, cranberries are so tart that they are usually heavily sweetened in commercial juices and in dried cranberries. High levels of sugars added to the juices and to the dried fruit promote poor colon health, rather than protect against UTIs. However, health/natural food stores sell unsweetened cranberry-juice concentrate, which can be diluted with water. Some cranberry juices are mixed with juices from sweet fruits. For purposes of urinary tract health, such dilution is inefficient. However, dried cranberries sweetened with fruit juice may be useful. Also, blueberries, which have similar beneficial qualities, offer an alternative choice.

The same compound that helps reduce UTIs may also benefit the teeth. According to Ervin I. Weiss, D.M.D., of Tel Aviv University in Israel, the polyphenols in unsweetened cranberry juice help prevent plaque on teeth by preventing the adherence of bacteria. Plaque formation is an early step in cavity development.

Weiss tested the effects of cranberry-juice extract on various species of *Streptococcus* and *Actinomyces*, the main bacteria known to cause cavities. He tested the extract with other species, too. Weiss found that the cranberry extract prevented the clumping together of 58 percent of the bacterial combinations tested. If the same effect could be produced on teeth, it might reduce the formation of dental plaque. Weiss reported that, unfortunately, the widely consumed commercial cranberry juice cocktail is not suited for oral-hygiene purposes; the high levels of sweetener(s) added promote plaque accumulation and caries development.

An additional value of cranberry juice was reported as early as 1964. In hospitals and nursing homes, urine odors can be a problem. The odor is caused by alkalinization and fermentation of foods in the intestinal tract. Cranberry juice increases urine acidity by reducing bacterial action and fermentation. Tests showed a positive decrease in urine odor within hours after patients drank cranberry juice. In dietary tests in two institutions, urine odor decreased significantly in patients during five days of cranberry-juice consumption. When the juice was not served, the urine odor returned to previous high levels.

Native American women used cranberry juice to dye rugs and blankets. Currently, food-processing companies use cranberry pigment as a natural food color. The ice-cream chain Baskin-Robbins uses buffered cranberry concentrate to add visual appeal to some of its ice-cream products.

Due to the antimicrobial activity of cranberry, an extract of the fruit is produced and made available to processors of foods, beverages, and nutritional supplements. Reportedly, the cranberry extract is thirty-two times more potent in inhibiting *E. coli* growth than its nearest competitor. Its resistance to many other bacteria and viruses makes it an effective preservative for foods that otherwise would spoil quickly due to microbial growth.

Raspberries

Both red and black raspberries contain antioxidants. Ellagic acid, quercetin glycosides, anthocyanins, and flavonol have all been identified as beneficial components of raspberries.

If you plan to plant raspberry canes in your garden, this information may interest you. Two popular summer-bearing cultivars are Lauren and Killarney, and two popular autumn-bearing ones are Heritage and Caroline. They all contain varying amounts of beta-carotene, fat-soluble vitamins A and E, water-soluble vitamin C, folic acid, and dietary fiber. However, in terms of antioxidant qualities, the Caroline cultivar is a clear winner.

In tests comparing the cultivars, Caroline was generally highest in nutrients. It was 20 percent higher in beta-carotene, 27 to 43 percent higher in vitamin A, 16 to 77 percent higher in vitamin E, and 25 to 48 percent higher in vitamin C, compared to the other raspberry cultivars tested. Also, the Caroline cultivar was higher overall in antioxidant content. Caroline had 47 percent more ORAC units than Lauren or Killarney, and 65 percent more ORAC units than the average of two Heritage fall-bearing red-raspberry samples tested. The Caroline cultivar had 2,130 ORAC units per 100 grams (g). By comparison, blueberries contain 2,400 units/g; and strawberries, 1,540 units/g. Research has suggested that 10 grams of freeze-dried Caroline red raspberries might provide 40 to 66 percent of the 3,000 to 5,000 ORAC units recommended for daily intake.

Red raspberries have been shown to reduce tumor activity in rats. Clinical studies conducted at the Hollings Cancer Center in Charleston, South Carolina, showed that ellagic acid in red raspberries was an effective anticarcinogen and antitumor initiator.

Other investigators studied the health benefits of red raspberry juice. Drs. Angelika Rommel and Ronald E. Wrolstad at Oregon State University reported that the phenolic content of concentrated red raspberry juice offers health benefits. The researchers used high-performance liquid chromatography to measure flavonol in the concentrate. They found that commercial samples varied greatly in their flavonol content. They suggested that two products with the lowest amount of quercetin glycosides might have been adulterated, because they also had low levels of flavonol, anthocyanin, and ellagic acid. Let the buyer beware! Choose whole raspberries rather than the concentrated juice. Also, because of the tartness of the concentrate, the product likely contains added sweetener(s).

Black raspberries also have been investigated for their health properties. Laura Ann Kresty and her colleagues at the College of Medicine of Ohio

State University in Columbus treated rats with a known cancer-causing chemical that induces esophageal cancer. Then, the researchers added freeze-dried black raspberries to the rats' feed. The rats on a diet containing 5 percent black raspberries developed 38.7 percent fewer esophageal tumors than the control group, which did not have berries added to the feed. Another group on a diet of 10 percent black raspberries developed 48.9 percent fewer esophageal tumors. The researchers concluded that the ellagic acid present in black raspberries was the main factor in preventing esophageal tumors in the rats. Berries are especially rich in ellagic acid. This antioxidant is also found in various other fruits and nuts.

SOME FAVORITE FRUITS

Some fruits such as apples and bananas are abundantly available year-round. Others such as cherries are seasonal treats.

Apples

"Increasing dietary consumption of fresh apples—with the skins on—provides additional phytochemicals that have a long-term health benefit and may prevent or reduce the risk of some chronic diseases," reported Chang Y. Lee, a food chemist in the Department of Food Science and Technology at the New York State Agricultural Experiment Station in Geneva, New York. (*Journal of Agricultural and Food Chemistry*, 2003; 3)

British researchers, both at King's College in London and at the University of Southampton, reported that people who ate at least two apples weekly had a 22 to 32 percent lower risk of developing asthma than people who ate fewer apples. The investigators' conclusions, which were based on studies with nearly 1,500 adults, suggested that the flavonoids in apples may reduce asthmatic inflammation through an antioxidant, antiallergenic, or anti-inflammatory response. (*American Journal of Respiratory and Critical Care Management*, 15 Nov 2001)

Other scientists at Nottingham University found that apples can promote healthy lungs, and alleviate several lung diseases and breathing disorders such as asthma. Of more than 2,600 adults with lung complaints, those who had the greatest lung capacity ate more than five apples weekly. The flavonoid quercetin, found in apples, was singled out as the antioxidant likely to protect the lungs from cigarette smoke and other environmental pollutants.

In May 2001, good news for men came from the Mayo Clinic in Rochester, Minnesota. Quercetin in apples (as well as in onions, tea, and red wine) may provide a new nonhormonal approach to prevent and treat prostate cancer. The study suggested that quercetin blocks hormonal activity of androgen (male sex hormone, primarily testosterone and a derivative of testosterone called dihydrotestosterone [DHT]), which has been associated with the development and progression of prostate cancer. (*Carcinogenesis*, March 2001)

The major antioxidant components in apples are polyphenols, contained mainly in the skin. They are quercetin and phloretin glycosides; chlorogenic acid; and epicatechin. Quercetin has proven helpful in reducing carcinogenic activity, inhibiting enzymatic activities associated with several types of tumor cells, enhancing the antiproliferation activity of anticancer agents, and inhibiting the growth of cells that have undergone tumorigenesis (tumor production).

Unfortunately, the skins of commercially grown apples are likely to contain pesticide residue, a waxed coating, and dirt that is trapped under the wax. For this reason, if you intend to eat the skins, it is important to obtain organically grown apples.

It is important, too, to eat the apple, rather than to drink apple juice. The extracted juice lacks the 3 to 4 grams of fiber (accounting for nearly 15 percent of the fiber recommended for daily intake) that is available in the whole apple.

Most of the fiber in apples is the soluble type that forms a gel when mixed with water. Insoluble fiber does not dissolve. Both soluble fiber and insoluble fiber are needed in the diet, but soluble fiber is less commonly available. When the soluble fiber gels, it collects and disposes of other compounds, such as bile salts, which contain cholesterol. Consuming adequate soluble fiber helps reduce the blood cholesterol level. Also, the gel slows down the flow of blood sugar from the digestive tract into the bloodstream, thus helping diabetics avoid swings in glucose levels. In addition to its soluble fiber, apples also contain insoluble fiber. Insoluble fiber consists of cellulose, which provides bulk and helps prevent constipation. Also, it helps eliminate toxins from the intestinal tract. These fibers are nonstarchy polysaccharides that human enzymes cannot break down and digest.

Another feature that makes apple juice less preferable to the whole apple is that the juice may be made from bruised and moldy fruit. Frequently, apple juice is contaminated by toxic molds such as patulin. Also, in recent years, there have been disease outbreaks from consumption of unpasteurized apple juice contaminated with pathogens such as *E. coli 0157:H7*.

The substitution of apple juice for milk to be given young children is a practice that has been criticized strongly by some pediatricians. In terms of nutrients, apple juice is not an adequate milk replacement. Additionally, the practice of giving a bottle of apple juice to infants at night has been deplored by some dentists. The natural sugar contained in the juice, especially in the acidic environment of apple juice, can lead to cavity formation in teeth. This is especially true if the juice is retained in the mouth of a sleeping infant.

Thus, for a number of reasons, eating the whole fruit—in this case, an apple—is preferable to drinking the juice. However, the apple is not particularly noteworthy for its content of vitamins and minerals. Other common fruits (and vegetables) are far better sources. Apples make only modest contributions. They contain about 13 percent of the RDA (recommended daily allowance) of vitamin C for adults, and about eight percent of the RDA for potassium.

Apples are more valuable for their antioxidant constituents. "Scientists are interested in isolated single compounds such as vitamin C, vitamin E, and beta-carotene to see if they exhibit antioxidant or anticancer benefits," noted Rui Hai Liu, Ph.D., assistant professor of food science at Cornell University. "It turns out," Liu continued, "that none of those work alone to reduce cancer. It's the combination of flavonoids and polyphenols doing the work." (*Stagnito's New Product Magazine,* June 2001)

Not all apples are equal in their antioxidant activity. Among different apple cultivars, those showing the highest activity are Northern Spy, Liberty, Crispin, Delicious, and Fuji; medium activity, Idared, Jonagold, Gala, Freedom, and McIntosh; and low activity, Empire, Ginger Gold, NY674, and Golden Delicious. Be guided by these findings when you are selecting apples for purchase or planting apple trees in your garden.

Bananas

This popular fruit is available throughout the year. Its sweetness and creamy texture appeal to people of all ages. Mashed banana is included among the first solid foods for infants; and the elderly, who may have problems chewing some foods due to poor dentition, favor bananas.

Individuals who are taking diuretics (water pills) consume bananas because they are a good source of potassium. Most diuretics deplete the body of potassium, and bananas, as well as other potassium-rich fruits, replenish this mineral in the body. Also, consuming an ample supply of potassium-rich foods appears to reduce the risk of stroke. One medium-sized banana (approximately 4 ounces) supplies about 450 milligrams (mg) of potassium, which is nearly one-fourth of the RDA of 2,000 mg.

In addition to potassium, one medium-sized banana supplies about 10 mg of vitamin C and about 33 mg of magnesium. Women need approximately 320 mg of magnesium daily; men, about 420 mg.

About 0.1 mg of vitamin B components, such as riboflavin (vitamin B_2) and thiamine (vitamin B_1), are provided in one banana. This sounds like a very small amount, but recommended daily intakes of these vitamins also are very small: riboflavin, 1.1 mg for women and 1.3 mg for men; thiamine, 1.1 mg for women and 1.2 mg for men.

One banana supplies about 3 grams of fiber. The recommended daily intake is between 20 and 25 grams of fiber daily. So, like apples, bananas are a good source of fiber.

If you buy green bananas, you can hasten the ripening process by putting the bananas in a tightly closed brown paper bag and storing it at room temperature. The slightly bitter starchiness of an unripe banana converts to fruit sugar when it ripens. The skin of a ripe banana has no green coloration but begins to develop some black specks. At this stage, the banana is ready to be eaten.

When red-skinned bananas are available, they are special treats. They ripen very slowly. When ripe, they are particularly sweet and have an exceptionally creamy texture.

Cherries

Many cherries are grown in the state of Michigan, so it is fitting that many of the health benefits of cherries are being studied at the University of Michigan at East Lansing. Some of the projects are funded by the Cherry Marketing Institute (CMI), a trade organization, along with the Michigan State University (MSU) Agriculture Experiment Station and a consortium of Midwestern universities known as the Midwest Advanced Food Manufacturing Alliance. Naturally, all groups are interested in promoting the benefits of cherries.

Tart red cherries have powerful antioxidants and anti-inflammatory properties. They help in the prevention of heart disease and cancer, and they relieve the pain of arthritis and gout. By strengthening blood vessel walls, the antioxidants may prevent varicose veins.

Muralee Nair, Ph.D., associate professor with the Bioactive Natural Products section in the Department of Horticulture at Michigan State University, in cooperation with the Natural Food Safety and Toxicology Center at MSU, has been investigating the properties of tart red cherries. At least seventeen compounds with antioxidant activity in the cherries have been identified. The three that provide the bright red pigment are especially strong antioxidants. Nair's analysis showed that these antioxidants were stronger than vitamins C and E, as well as some synthetic antioxidants used by food processors.

Other research at MSU studies cherry's effects on arthritis. It appears that the anthocyanins in cherries offer positive results for arthritic sufferers. The anthocyanins in tart red cherries were up to ten times more effective in relieving joint pains, inflammation, and painful conditions such as gout, compared to commonly used medications such as aspirin and ibuprofen. Also, the red cherries were found to have substantial amounts of melatonin, another naturally occurring antioxidant that helps to regulate sleep patterns.

The anthocyanins appear to inhibit cyclooxygenase-1 and -2. These enzymes, which are involved in inflammation, are targeted by anti-inflammatory drugs. The anthocyanins also prevent oxidative damage caused by oxygen and free radicals. Thus, anthocyanins have been dubbed "Mother Nature's all-natural chemotherapy agents."

Some health benefits were observed in cherry growers. Many of them consume about six times as many cherries as the average American. A survey, conducted by CMI in collaboration with Wirthlin Worldwide, a national opinion research organization, found that cherry growers have significantly fewer signs of heart disease and a lower risk of cancer than the general population.

Laboratory assays of tart red cherries suggest that a person who eats about twenty tart cherries obtains approximately 12 to 25 milligrams of anthocyanins. Such a daily intake might be sufficient to achieve the antioxidant and anti-inflammatory benefits derived from cherries.

The antioxidant property of cherries is being utilized by some food processors. Spoilage of stored raw ground beef is reduced by adding cherries to the mixture. In one study, after raw hamburgers were stored with added cherries in a refrigerator for four days, the meat contained less than half as much oxidized cholesterol as untreated meat. Previous research has suggested that oxidized cholesterol (especially LDL cholesterol) is more harmful to health than regular cholesterol.

The addition of cherries to raw hamburgers also reduces the formation of carcinogenic compounds that form when the meat is grilled. When cherries are mixed with hamburger meat, the harmful heterocyclic aromatic amines (HAAs) can be lowered by 70 percent. (*Journal of Agricultural and Food Chemistry*, Dec 1998)

The addition of 13 percent tart red cherries can serve as a fat substitute in hamburgers. The ground beef/cherry mixture, with 10 percent fat, has shown significantly better flavor in the cooked hamburgers. Food processors are exploring the possibility of adding cherries to other high-moisture foods.

A drawback in the use of cherries for these purposes in processed foods is that its addition to food is unconventional and, therefore, unsuspected by consumers. The addition of the cherries may provoke an allergic reaction. Although cherry allergy is uncommon, *any* food can be an allergen for some individuals.

Citrus Fruits

Many Americans drink orange juice religiously as part of breakfast. They feel comforted that the juice will provide enough vitamin C to take care of their daily needs. This concept has been fostered with aggressive promotion by trade organizations and citrus-growing states. By now, the reader of this book knows that it is better to eat the whole fruit, in this case the orange, than to drink the juice, and to vary fruit consumption from day to day.

Oranges and other citrus fruits are overrated in terms of their vitamin C content, which varies widely, depending on many factors. For example, there is a difference between the vitamin C content of navel oranges and that of Valencia oranges—and the exact levels of the vitamin within the two varieties change according to where the fruit is grown.

The vitamin C content of a citrus fruit also depends on the number of seeds in the fruit. The greater the number of seeds, the higher is the vitamin C content. Years ago, citrus fruit contained many seeds. Plant breeders have succeeded in reducing, or even eliminating, the seeds in currently grown varieties, purportedly for greater consumer appeal.

Shipping and storage conditions, and handling of the fruit in the home, are additional factors in vitamin C retention. After you purchase citrus fruits, transfer them to the crisper section of your refrigerator. The fruits will retain their vitamin C for a few weeks; after that, there will be a gradual decline. After washing, peeling and segmenting citrus fruit, it should be eaten promptly. Remember that as soon as you cut the fruit, expose it to heat, air, or light, or froth it in a blender, the fruit will suffer a decline in vitamin C.

A ten-year study of Florida-processed orange and grapefruit juices tested for their vitamin C content. Hyoung Lee and Gary Coates from the Florida Department of Citrus at Lake Alfred, Florida, analyzed more than 2,200 samples of orange and grapefruit juices made by twenty-one Florida processors. The samples included juices from frozen concentrates (from which water has been extracted from the concentrate), juices from concentrates (to which the extracted water has been restored), and pasteurized juices. The vitamin C content varied considerably once taken to market, depending on the types of containers used and the market's conditions. (*Journal of Agricultural Food Chemistry*, 1997; 45: 2550)

In earlier studies, Florida-grown Tahiti limes (Persian) were analyzed for their vitamin C content. Tahiti limes are harvested year-round in Florida. The concentration of vitamin C was found to be greatest in May and June, and lowest in February and March. The vitamin level was higher for small limes than for large ones. Also, the vitamin C levels varied from grove to grove, because the soil fertility probably varied.

Most studies of citrus fruits only measure ascorbic acid (vitamin C) content. However, Richard R. Streiff, M.D., at the College of Medicine, University of Florida, measured folates (folic acid and folacin) in citrus fruits. Streiff considered 50–100 micrograms (mcg) of folate daily as an acceptable intake for adults. He found nearly a twofold difference among various types of citrus fruits. The juice of Valencia oranges provided 28 mcg of folate per 100 milliliters (ml); Parson Brown, 36 mcg/ml; Hamlin, 31 mcg/ml; Murcott, 22 mcg/ml; Pineapple orange, 41 mcg/ml; Dancy tangerine, 21 mcg/ml; and Orlando tangelo, 15 mcg/ml. (*American Journal of Clinical Nutrition*, Dec 1971; 24 [2]: 1390–1392)

Although in the past great emphasis was placed on the value of citrus fruit for its contribution of vitamin C, more recently, attention has been turned to its beneficial phytochemicals. Monoterpenes are phytochemicals present in citrus fruits. One monoterpene is D-limonene, which can stimulate the development of detoxification enzymes that inhibit mammary tumor growth. In experiments, D-limonene was capable of causing regression of carcinoma in rat mammary tumors.

In test-tube experiments at the University of Western Ontario, Canada, Kenneth K. Carroll, Ph.D., director of the Centre for Human Nutrition, found that naringenin, a flavonoid in grapefruit juice, was almost eight times more potent in inhibiting cell growth than genistein, an estrogenlike flavonoid in soy that also inhibits cell growth. However, naringenin was less effective than genistein in slowing the growth of breast cancer cells that depend on estrogen for growth.

Carroll reported that citrus fruits may significantly delay the growth of breast cancer cells, as well as reduce LDL cholesterol. In the breast cancer study, the researchers tested the ability of orange and grapefruit juices, and their constituent flavonoids, to inhibit human breast cancer cells injected into mice. Compared to the animals that drank water, those that drank orange or grapefruit juice developed only half as many tumors, and the cancer metastasized (spread to other parts of the body) half as quickly. The group consuming only flavonoids also had fewer tumors, but not as few as the groups consuming the citrus juices. This finding suggests that other active components in the fruits, in addition to the flavonoids, helped reduce the number of tumors.

An unanticipated effect observed in this study was that cholesterol levels declined dramatically in the animals given the citrus juices. To study this unexpected finding, the researchers extended the work, using rabbits. Orange juice appeared to be especially effective in reducing LDL cholesterol in these animals. In rabbits fed orange juice, LDL cholesterol levels declined by 43 percent, and in those fed grapefruit juice, levels declined by 32 percent.

In two rat trials, orange juice again outperformed grapefruit juice in lowering LDL cholesterol. However, in all studies looking at actions against cancer and cholesterol, naringenin in grapefruits surpassed hesperidin, a flavonoid in oranges. Carroll hoped to conduct future studies on the cancer-inhibiting effects of oranges and tangerines in mice injected with human cancer cells.

In follow-up studies, the researchers tested tangerines and other citrus fruits. The most potent inhibitors of cancer cell growth were two flavonoids from tangerines: tangeretin and nobiletin. Each one of these flavonoids was about 250 times more potent than genistein in estrogen-sensitive cells and five to nine times more potent in estrogen-dependent cancerous cells. When delivered together or along with other fruit flavonoids, these two tangerine flavonoids were even more potent. Also, they seemed to increase the effectiveness of tamoxifen (a drug used in breast cancer treatment).

At the USDA's Horticultural Research Laboratory at Fort Pierce in Florida, Agricultural Research Service investigators identified some antioxidant bioflavonoids in citrus fruits that may help the body resist carcinogens. Hesperidin, the most abundant bioflavonoid in oranges, inhibited the P450 IB1 enzyme from metabolizing precarcinogens, thus reducing the chance that the body could convert these substances into cancer-producing substances.

In the early 1990s, Dr. David Bailey, a pharmacologist at the Victoria Hospital and University of Western Ontario in London, Ontario, noted that grapefruit juice helped the body absorb certain drugs into the blood. Oddly, orange juice did not. Dr. Bailey and his colleagues explored this observation, believing that this finding might have practical applications.

Bailey gave one group of volunteers felodipine (at the time, an experimental drug used to treat high blood pressure and later marketed as Plendil) with grapefruit juice and alcohol. Another group of volunteers took the same drug with grapefruit juice, but without alcohol. Then, the researchers tested the blood levels of felodipine in both groups. The amount of the drug found in the bloodstream of the volunteers was several times higher than the level that had been reported by the scientists who had worked on developing the drug. The difference was, in their experiments, they had used orange juice.

The puzzled researchers wondered if grapefruit juice somehow had interfered with the laboratory testing system. After much experimentation, they found that the grapefruit juice was the one factor causing the higher-than-expected level of felodipine in the bloodstream. A customary dose of the drug, taken with grapefruit juice, increased *fivefold* in the bloodstream, compared to the same amount of the drug taken with water. Whether the grapefruit juice was freshly squeezed or frozen did not affect results.

Enzymes in the body destroy about 85 percent of a drug—such as the calcium channel blocker felodipine—as it is being absorbed, allowing only about 15 percent of the drug to enter circulating blood. More of the drug is broken down as it continues to pass through the blood and the liver. Apparently, some component of grapefruit juice, which is not present in orange juice, was inhibiting the enzymes from functioning and was allowing for much greater drug absorption. Naringenin was identified as the component.

In another study, grapefruit juice taken with nifedipine (a calcium channel blocker known as Procardia or Adalat and used for heart and blood pressure conditions) boosted the drug's availability to the body by *134 percent.*

Dr. Bailey and his associates began, systematically, to test other drugs to learn how many might be affected by grapefruit juice. They discovered that other drugs, too, could have their potencies altered by grapefruit juice. (*Lancet*, 29 Feb 1991)

Originally, the discovery of grapefruit's effect on some medications was regarded as potentially beneficial. However, gradually, the finding came to be viewed with concern. It was learned that grapefruit juice could increase the concentration of such medications dramatically and lead to dangerous, or even deadly, abnormalities of heart rhythm. Signs and symptoms included heart palpitations, dizziness, fainting, chest discomfort, and shortness of breath.

The popular, nonsedating antihistamine terfenadine (Seldane and Seldane-D) is a medication known to interact with grapefruit and have potentially serious consequences. Naringenin, as well as other flavonoids present in grapefruit, interferes with the function of a critical liver enzyme, CYP-

3A4. Normally, this enzyme would process terfenadine or other drugs. With naringenin's interference with CYP-3A4, the drug level might reach an excessively high and dangerously toxic level in the blood. If this occurs, individuals could experience a serious change in heart rhythm known as "torsade de pointes." Another nonsedating antihistamine, astemizole (Hismanal), should not be taken with grapefruit juice.

Findings from these studies suggest that if you are taking certain medications that require liquid for swallowing pills, do *not* use grapefruit juice as the liquid. Use water. If you use an over-the-counter antacid drug, avoid drinking orange juice, as well as grapefruit juice; these drugs contain aluminum, and undesirable high-aluminum absorption can result from the acidity of citrus fruits, combined with the antacid.

Grapes

Grapes are a popular fruit, of which there are numerous varieties. Available throughout the year, grapes have been shown to confer numerous health benefits. Grapes have high amounts of ellagic acid, one of the beneficial phenolic compounds that appears to lower cancer risk. Also, new research has shown components of grapes to contain the powerful antioxidant called resveratrol.

Currently, there is much interest in muscadine grapes, which are native to America. They are also known as bullace grapes, scuppernongs, and southern fox grapes. At the Small Fruit Research Laboratory in Poplarville, Mississippi, researchers from the Agricultural Research Service, in collaboration with scientists from Mississippi State University, found that the skin, pulp, and seeds of muscadine grapes have high levels of resveratrol. This is exciting news because, to date, this valuable naturally occurring substance had been found mainly in the skins of red grapes. This finding also could help promote muscadines as eating grapes and for jams and jellies. Only about half of all muscadines are processed into juice; the remainder is considered waste. While some of this remainder is added to low-value animal feed, the rest poses an environmental disposal problem.

In recent years, a component of resveratrol has created much enthusiasm among investigators. It is a hydroxylated stilbene, found especially in the skins of red grapes. It is found in other foods, too, including mulberry and peanut.

Among resveratrol's many characteristics, it has been found to act as an antioxidant and antimutagen, and to mediate anti-inflammatory effects. In carcinogen-treated mouse mammary glands, resveratrol inhibited the development of new tumors. It also inhibited tumor growth in a mouse skin-cancer model. These observations suggest that resveratrol may be a potential cancer-preventative agent in humans.

At first, attention was given to resveratrol in red wines. In 1992, Leroy L. Creasy, Ph.D., professor of pomology at New York State College of Agriculture and Life Sciences at Cornell University in Ithaca, New York, made international headlines by reporting that resveratrol, present in red wine, might lower cholesterol levels in humans. Generally, concentrations of resveratrol are found highest in red wines, which are made from grapes fermented in their skins. By far, Bordeaux wine showed the highest level of resveratrol. To date, how much resveratrol is needed by humans to lower cholesterol levels has not been established.

Originally, Creasy's interest in resveratrol was due to his work as a pomologist (a scientist who works with fruits). Resveratrol is a naturally occurring antifungal agent present in grape skins that protects the fruit. He found that resveratrol was released from the skin during fermentation—hence, the connection with wine.

After the publicity was generated regarding the potential cardiac benefits of red wine, some drinkers clamored to know if white wine yielded similar benefits. In making white wine, the grape skins are removed before fermentation. For this reason, white wine contains very little resveratrol.

Nonalcoholic imbibers were interested to learn whether red grapes and juices made from them yielded benefits similar to those of red wine. To answer this question, Creasy and his colleagues continued their investigations of resveratrol with grape juices.

Although in processing grapes into juices, the products are not fermented, Creasy discovered that the grapes do release resveratrol as the juices are heated in processing. Creasy analyzed purple grape juice from eighteen samples taken from three different regions of the country, and he found that the juices contained *more resveratrol than in 60 percent of the red wines tested.* The juices consistently registered 100–150 micrograms per liter (mcg/l). Creasy termed this finding "amazingly constant." In contrast, the level of resveratrol in various red wines was unpredictable. Some samples had as much as 550 mcg/l and others had undetectable levels. Creasy concluded that purple grape juice may be more reliable than wine in providing a beneficial level of resveratrol.

The processing of juice is less variable than the wine-making process. Also, purple grape juice usually is made from a single grape variety, Concord grape. Wine may be made from numerous grape varieties. Creasy's earlier work looking at resveratrol's ability to combat fungal diseases led him to find that disease-resistant varieties of grapes produce much more resveratrol than the disease-susceptible varieties.

Studies from various places corroborate the early findings that purple grape juice has the same effect as red wine in reducing the risk of heart disease. In Japan, researchers working with rats found that resveratrol lowered cholesterol and reduced the rate of platelet aggregation (clumping). This condition is associated with arterial damage and heart disease.

At Georgetown University Medical Center in Washington, D.C., investigators found that alcohol, only at intoxicating levels, inhibits blood clots. With purple grape juice, platelets clotted about 30 percent less than in controls and released three times more nitric oxide. Nitric oxide is a chemical that dilates blood vessels and acts as a powerful clotting inhibitor, thereby preventing platelet aggregation. These actions reduce the likelihood that blood clots will block arteries and lead to heart attacks.

In 1997, both a laboratory experiment with monkeys and a clinical trial with humans, conducted at the University of Wisconsin, suggested that grape juice might protect against heart attacks. The grape juice inhibited blood platelets from aggregating and reduced the risk of blocked arteries. What made these two studies different from those mentioned above was that the value of grape juice was compared to aspirin, a compound used to prevent blood-platelet aggregation. An 8-ounce dosage of grape juice, given daily, reduced platelet aggregation both in monkeys and humans as effectively as aspirin.

This study was extended the following year. John Folts, Ph.D., director of the Coronary Thrombosis Research Laboratory at the University of Wisconsin's Medical School, measured the degree of aggregation by platelets in the blood of five men and five women. Then, he had the ten volunteers drink 2 cups of purple grape juice daily for a week, after which he took new measurements of their blood. The grape juice had reduced platelet aggregation by an average of 84 percent. This reduction was greater than any that had ever been reported for aspirin. Folts substituted grapefruit and orange juices for the purple grape juice, but these juices showed no effect on platelet aggregation.

The following year, Folts's ongoing research suggested that purple grape juice may delay the oxidation of LDL cholesterol among people with coronary artery disease, even in individuals who have already taken vitamin E. At a scientific session of the American College of Cardiology, Folts said, "We know that the oxidation of LDL is a key contributor to the development of atherosclerosis—which is a buildup of plaque in the coronary artery."

A number of different naturally occurring flavonoids function as antioxidants, anti-inflammatory agents, and inhibitors of platelet aggregation. In addition, flavonoids are capable of protecting the arterial wall from damage and, thereby, may inhibit atherosclerotic development. Red and purple grapes contain these constituents.

In recent years, attention has been given to the seeds in grapes. At Creighton University in Omaha, Nebraska, a powerful antioxidant was discovered in red grape seeds. The substance activin was reported to neutralize and inhibit free radicals in the brains and livers of mice. As an antioxidant, activin was up to seven times more potent than vitamins C or E, or beta-carotene.

Elsewhere, research with grape seed showed that the high potency of flavonoid extracts, especially catechins and proanthocyanidins, provide antioxidant and cardiovascular benefits. Grape seed extract is reported to demonstrate strong protective effects against microvascular disorders, atherosclerosis, cataracts, gastric ulcers, and joint inflammation. These findings suggest that one should regard grapes as "whole foods"—by chewing and consuming the seeds as well as the grapes.

Melons

Among the many melons grown, watermelon is one of the favorites. It is thirst quenching in hot weather. Low in calories, it is a boon to dieters. It also tastes good. Although watermelon consists of much water, it does contain valuable nutrients. According to the USDA's nutrient database, 2 cups of diced watermelon (about 10 ounces) has only 100 calories. Of this amount, watermelon contains almost 31 milligrams (mg) of vitamin C; nearly 1,200 IU of vitamin A; about 0.5 mg of pyridoxine (vitamin B_6); and about 0.25 mg of thiamine (vitamin B_1). It contains more than 370 mg of potassium and more than 35 mg of magnesium. Watermelon also contains almost 0.2 grams of lysine, an essential amino acid.

Beyond the nutrients in watermelon is its content of the carotenoid lycopene. As previously mentioned, there is much interest in this carotenoid, especially because it was found that the body absorbs increased amounts of lycopene from cooked tomatoes. (See Chapter 1 for a discussion of raw vs. cooked vegetables.)

New chemical analyses were conducted by nutritionists Beverly A. Clevidence and Alison J. Edwards at the USDA's Agricultural Research Service Laboratory in Beltsville, Maryland. They recruited twenty-three healthy men and women for three separate three-week trial sessions. In each phase, the scientists administered all the food eaten by the volunteers.

During the first session, each individual ate a diet low in lycopene. During the next session, the diet was supplemented daily with 3 cups of watermelon juice that contained 20 milligrams (mg) of lycopene.

In the third session, half of the recruits consumed daily tomato-juice servings containing 20 mg of lycopene; the other half received enough watermelon juice daily to provide 40 mg of lycopene. The tomato juice was a canned, heat-processed product. The watermelon was uncooked, frozen juice. In both groups, blood levels of lycopene increased to twice the amount measured at the beginning of the experiment. This was the first study to show that the body takes up lycopene from watermelon.

Chemical analysis by USDA scientists showed that the red pigment of watermelon can have about 40 percent more lycopene than an equivalent weight of uncooked tomato. A second analysis showed that the lycopene in raw watermelon is more available to the body than lycopene in raw tomato.

Pomegranates

This seasonal fruit—literally "apple with many seeds"—has been eaten for as long as 5,000 to 6,000 years. It was among the first fruits to be cultivated, and its origins are thought to have been in the Middle East, in the area of present-day Syria and Iran. The fruit, being hardy, was transported by caravans and spread to Afghanistan, India, Egypt, and China.

The pomegranate was important in ancient Greek mythology and early literature. The Bible makes several references to the pomegranate. With the pomegranate's graceful shape, it was used as a motif on the skirts of high priests' robes, as decoration for Solomon's Temple, and carved in the capitals of stone pillars in Asian temples. The Crusaders brought the pomegranate back to medieval Europe, and the conquistadors spread it to the New World. Not only was the pomegranate enjoyed as an edible fruit, but it was used medicinally, as a cathartic, astringent, antidiarrheal, and anthelmintic (agent that protects against intestinal parasites).

With recent interest in the values of fruits beyond their nutrient offerings, the pomegranate has been found to benefit vascular health. It is a good source of antioxidants, especially ellagic acid, flavonoids, and polyphenols.

The image of the pomegranate is dual. Because of the hundreds of seeds contained in a single fruit, the pomegranate has been a symbol of fertility. However, the pomegranate has been regarded, too, as an antifertility agent. Investigations have shown that this fruit contains weak estrogens (oestrone, alpha-estradiol, and estriol), genistein, daidzein, and coumestrol, as well as testosterone.

To prepare a pomegranate, remove the leathery rind. Try not to cut into the seeds. Then, carefully, peel away the white segments that encase the seeds. Separate the seeds and eat them intact. These jewel-like seeds also make an attractive addition to fruit salads. Refrigerate unused seeds in a tightly closed jar and use them within a week or two.

SOME FAVORITE DRIED FRUITS

The portability of dried fruits makes them popular for snacking. However, due to their intense concentration of fruit sugars, the consumption of dried fruits should be limited. Also, dried fruits stick to the teeth. If you eat them, promptly reach for the floss and toothbrush!

Raisins

Raisins are among the popular dried fruits. They contribute dietary fiber, vitamins, and minerals such as potassium, phosphorus, copper, and iron to the diet. Also, among the antioxidants, they contain flavonoids such as catechin and quercetin.

A USDA study on antioxidants at Tufts University showed that a snack of 100 grams of raisins provides more than 2,800 ORAC units. (See "The Top-Scoring Fruits for Antioxidants" on page 41.) Also, $\frac{1}{4}$ cup of raisins contains about 1.5 grams of inulin, a prebiotic. Prebiotics are nutrients utilized by beneficial organisms, typically in the form of indigestible oligosaccharides that arrive in the colon intact, to be metabolized by the resident bacterial flora. Prebiotics promote beneficial bacteria in the gut. In contrast, a probiotic is a live microbial food ingredient that has a beneficial effect on human health. The probiotic bacteria aid the immune system to ward off foodborne pathogens. Also, they lower the pH in the colon, which may help lower the risk of colon cancer.

Prunes

Prunes are among the most commonly used dried fruits. They have suffered from a poor image. As early as the 1960s, a leading motivational expert, Ernest Dichter, Ph.D., warned the prune industry that its product had unpleasant associations in the public mind, such as constipation, devitalization, dried-out spinsters, and the wrinkles of old age. Dichter urged the industry to revamp the image and present prunes as the juicy California wonder fruit, with photographs on prune-juice containers giving the fruit more of a purple than a brown hue. The prunes remained unchanged but miraculously had acquired a new persona.

More recently, once again, the prune was reinvented. In June 2000, the U.S. Food and Drug Administration (FDA) granted the California Prune Board (CPB) permission to use the term "dried plums" as an alternative to "prunes." CPB officials requested the name change after their research had indicated that the public views the name "dried plum" more favorably than "prune." CPB hopes that the new name will attract new consumers from its target audience, women aged thirty-five to fifty years.

Recently, dried plums (a.k.a. prunes) have been found to be effective as a food-safety ingredient, at a time when the issue of food safety looms large. Daniel Fung, Ph.D., at the Department of Animal Sciences and Industry at Kansas State University in Manhattan, Kansas, conducted extensive research on the ability of certain constituents in food to inhibit foodborne contaminants. Professor Fung discovered effective microbial inhibitors in dried plum purée and in fresh plum juice. Using ground beef, the constituents were tested for their ability to inhibit the growth of major pathogens. Both the dried plum purée and fresh plum juice significantly inhibited *E. coli 0157:H7*, *Salmonella typhimurium*, *Listeria monocytogenes*, *Yersinia enterocolitica*, and *Staphylococcus aureus*. Using a 3 percent level, by weight, of dried plum purée, Professor Fung achieved up to a 99 percent kill rate for some of these pathogens in ground meats.

An additional benefit of dried plum purée was found in its effect on "warmed-over flavor" (a term used by food technologists to describe a flavor degradation) caused by lipid oxidation in precooked pork sausage. The oxidation of the fat leads to rancidity, which is toxic. In studies done by Jimmy T. Keeton, Ph.D., in the Department of Animal Sciences at Texas A&M University in College Station, Texas, dried plum purée was more effective in preventing lipid oxidation in the meat than the commonly used synthetic antioxidants, BHT and BHA (butylated hydroxytoluene and butylated hydroxyanisole).

As a result of these studies, dried plum purée is being added to many precooked, heat-and-serve prepared meat and poultry food products, including beef patties, Italian sausages, hot dogs, turkey patties, chicken sausages, sauces, and home-meal replacement (HMR) entrées. Although the addition of dried plum purée to meats may offer benefits of safety and flavor, they have the same drawbacks as when cherry purée, for similar reasons, is added to meat. Consumers will not expect the fruit purée in the meat and may unknowingly expose themselves to a food allergen. (See section on cherries earlier in this chapter.)

BUYING AND STORING FRUITS

Some fresh fruits such as bananas and apples are available in food stores year-round. Others such as fresh peaches and cherries are seasonal. Some fruits such as apples, kiwis, pineapple, and citrus fruits are quite durable and will keep well if you store them in a cool, dry place. Others such as fresh raspberries are highly perishable, and you need to refrigerate and use them promptly.

Unripe green bananas may turn yellow and ripen with astonishing rapidity if you store them in a warm room. On the other hand, unripe pears take their time to reach a good stage of ripeness. There seems to be a fine line between the peak of ripeness and a state of mold or other signs of deterioration in some fruits. Many factors need to be considered when you purchase fruits: Do you plan to use the fruit immediately, or in the near future? Do you have enough storage room in the refrigerator for a bag of grapefruit? Do you have time to prepare a pomegranate? Will the melon be ripe when you plan to serve it to guests later this week? Is it wise to buy fresh strawberries, knowing that you will be away from home for a few days? These, and many other decisions, need to be made every time you shop for fresh fruit.

Some fruits, such as melons and bananas, store well at room temperature. Other fresh fruits, such as peaches, nectarines, apricots, plums, and grapes, need refrigeration.

Wash all fruits just before you plan to eat them. Advance washing, before refrigeration, hastens their deterioration needlessly. When you do wash fresh fruits, remove the surface dirt and contaminants from bird droppings or pathogens transmitted from fruit growers, pickers, or handlers. It is difficult to wash clusters of grapes. You can wash them more thoroughly by removing the grapes from the stems. Place the individual grapes in a colander and rinse thoroughly. Similarly, rinse berries in a colander, and remove any leaves, debris, or moldy berries.

Cut fruits just before you plan to use them. This practice prevents oxidation, seen in browning, and loss of vitamin C.

It is prudent to wash *all* fruits prior to use, even those with thick rinds. There are cases reported of people who were made ill by pathogens on the rinds of cantaloupe. When the unwashed cantaloupes were cut open, the pathogens were transferred by the cutting knives from the rinds to the edible interior pulp.

Although the skins of apples and pears have nutrients, they may have residues of pesticides. Unless such fruits are grown organically or biodynamically, it is best to peel such treated fruits.

You can increase your fruit consumption quite easily. Besides the perennial favorites, many other fruits can be added to the diet. The variety of available fruits is now richer than ever. Presently, thanks to a rich cultural mix and better transport and storage facilities, some markets now offer carambola (star fruit), plantain, papaya, mango, kiwi, and pawpaw. Newer introductions include, among others, passion fruit, pitahaya (dragon fruit), and tamarillo. Try new fruits whenever they are available, and enjoy.

Use fruits for desserts and snacks. Fruits and cheeses make simple, quick-to-prepare, and satisfying desserts. Take easy-to-transport fruits, such as an apple or a tangerine, for a between-meal snack. Out with the doughnut—in with the fruit!

CHAPTER 3

Wholesome
Whole Grains

*The protection seen with whole-grain consumption is much
greater than we would predict from the soluble-fiber content
alone. The whole is greater than the sum of its parts. Even when
we look at all the parts of whole grain that we know protect
against heart disease—vitamins, minerals, soluble fiber, stanols,
etc.—the protectiveness of whole-grain intake is greater than the
sum of the protection seen with all the pieces. It's more than
just fiber; it is the whole food, literally, the whole grain.*

—JOANNE L. SLAVIN, PROFESSOR OF NUTRITION, UNIVERSITY OF MINNESOTA, ST. PAUL, FROM THE
JOURNAL OF THE AMERICAN DIETETIC ASSOCIATION (JULY 2001)

"Today, Western man has revolutionized the production, storage, and distribution of his foods," bemoaned the late trace mineral expert, Henry A. Schroeder, M.D., in the book *Pollution, Profits, and Progress* (Stephen Greene Press, 1971). "He refines his wheat, serving about 30 percent of it as bran, germ, and raw flour to his domestic livestock, and saving for himself the purified white 70 percent that is flour . . . . He refines his rice until it is pure and white, serving the rich brown residues to animals, or discarding it." Schroeder concluded that "pure" food is not good food for humans, because the refinement process removes vitamins and minerals that are fed to livestock that thrive on them.

NUTRIENT LOSSES IN REFINED GRAIN

With the introduction of steel-rolling mills, which replaced the local grist mills, speedy, large-scale milling of white flour became possible. The grain was crushed rather than ground, which allowed the starchy portion of the flour to be separated from the germ and bran through sifting. The flour, without the fat from the germ, could be stored or shipped long distances without turning rancid. This gave the flour a long shelf life, which suited millers and bakers. Other grain fractions could be sold separately and profitably, including the bran, the germ, the "shorts" or "middlings," and the gluten. In the cities, bran could be used as horse feed or processed into ship biscuits (hardtack eaten on long voyages). In the countryside, bran was eaten by the rural population, or used in animal feed.

The milling operations impoverished the flour in a manner that even today the average consumer scarcely appreciates. By crushing the grain, the rolling mill destroys the cellular structure of the grain and alters its biological pattern. The rolling mill reduces both the quality and the quantity of the proteins. Good-quality proteins are removed with the germ and bran; only poor-quality protein remains in the refined flour. For example, the amino acids lysine and tryptophan, essential for growth, are reduced. Also, the balances of minerals are disturbed. For example, the ratio of potassium to magnesium is altered, as are the ratios of potassium to sodium, zinc to cadmium, and iron to zinc. The grain contains valuable unsaturated fatty acids and vitamin E, and in using the rolling mill, the grain loses about half of its fat content. Wheat germ, which is lost in the refinement process, is one of the richest sources of vitamin E.

The removal of the brown-colored wheat germ and bran allowed bakers to use a light-colored flour for their products. The white appearance and the lighter texture served the ever-growing appeal for whiteness and lightness in foods. The market demanded refined flour, sugar, salt, and milk.

To obtain "pure" white flour, Schroeder noted, Western man removes from wheat 60 percent of the calcium, 75 percent of the phosphorus, 85 percent of the magnesium, 77 percent of the potassium, and 77 percent of the sodium present in the original grain of wheat. Even more serious, according to Schroeder, is the loss of trace minerals: 50 percent of the chromium, 86 percent of the manganese, 76 percent of the iron, 89 percent of the cobalt, 68 percent of the copper, 78 percent of the zinc, and 48 percent of the molybdenum.

The vitamin losses that result from refining wheat are dramatic, too: 77 percent of thiamine (vitamin B_1), 80 percent of riboflavin (vitamin B_2), 81 percent of niacin (vitamin B_3), 72 percent of pyridoxine (vitamin B_6), and 86 percent of vitamin E. Other fractions of the vitamin B complex, such as biotin, inositol, folic acid, choline, and para-aminobenzoic acid (PABA), are all reduced.

In an attempt to make up for these lost minerals and vitamins (but not trace minerals), iron and a few vitamins are added to the flour in the so-called enrichment program, launched by the U.S. Department of Agriculture (USDA) in 1941. Although numerous nutrients are removed from the whole grain in converting it to refined flour, in the "enrichment" program only a few are added back.

In the case of adding back iron, the millers can decide which iron compound they use. They select iron compounds that will not impart an off-color or off-flavor to the flour when it is used by bakers. They are not necessarily iron compounds that are well absorbed in the human body. Also, when iron is restored, but zinc and copper are not, former ratios are lost. Also, when iron is restored in a greater amount than was originally present in the grain, it poses a threat to individuals with hemochromatosis, a disorder of iron accumulation. Yet, some have suggested *tripling* the amount of iron in flour; however, this is a questionable solution to iron-deficiency diseases, as too much iron can be toxic.

In recent years, it has been mandated that folic acid be added to flour, because the nutrient was found to be involved in embryonic and fetal nerve-cell formation. Adequate supplies of folic acid and other B-vitamin fractions are vital for pregnant women in order to prevent neural-tube defects, including spina bifida and anencephaly in the offspring. However, the synthesized folic acid added to flour is not as well absorbed and utilized as the folate form present in whole foods. Would it not be more sensible as an official policy to recommend the consumption of whole-grain flours, in which folic acid is a natural constituent?

The enrichment program breaks numerous relationships that exist between nutrients, including dependencies and antagonisms. An example is cadmium and zinc. Cadmium in the whole grain is not well absorbed in the body in the presence of zinc. Zinc is concentrated in the germ and bran of the whole grain, where it is held until needed to grow roots before the young plant can obtain it from the soil. Cadmium, on the other hand, is distributed throughout the grain. The result of removing the germ and bran, then, is that most of the zinc is removed, whereas the toxic cadmium remains in the grain. In the whole grain, cadmium's toxic effects are held in check by the zinc. However, the zinc is no longer available. The result is that the toxic cadmium remains unbuffered in the refined flour. (Sugar, too, in refining loses its supply of zinc, but the cadmium remains.)

REDISCOVERING WHOLE GRAINS

During the 1990s, much attention was given to identifying phytochemicals in vegetables and fruits. Ultimately, and overdue, by the late 1990s, some attention was directed to the beneficial roles of phytochemicals in whole grains. In conjunction with nutrients, phytochemicals in whole grains were found to contribute to health and disease prevention. Some of the discoveries paralleled those with vegetables and fruits.

Numerous studies have indicated that greater consumption of whole-grain products significantly reduces the risk of cancer, heart disease, stroke, digestive problems, obesity, and diabetic complications. However, only about 13 percent of Americans consume one or more servings of whole-grain products daily. (*Journal of the American Dietetics Association,* July 2001; 101 [71]: 780–785) In the revised 2005 *Dietary Guidelines for Americans,* the USDA recommended increased whole-grain consumption.

A focus on dietary fibers, especially soluble ones, has tended to overshadow the roles of whole grains in their contributions to a healthy diet. The constituent of dietary fiber is merely one factor. Whole grains, in contrast to refined flours made from them, provide complex carbohydrates, resistant starch (insoluble fiber and nondigestible carbohydrate), vitamins, minerals, and many antioxidants and phytochemicals. The weakly estrogenic phytoestrogens (plant-based estrogens) in some whole grains promote healthy vascular responses to stress. Phytic acid, found in high levels in whole grains, can chelate pro-oxidant metals such as lead, aluminum, cadmium, and mercury, and inhibit oxidative damage. (A chelator binds to the metal and excretes it from the body.) Whole-grain products require much chewing and have a higher satiety index than products made with refined grain flours. Vitamin E and selenium, which work in tandem, are especially high in whole grains. Also, whole grains lower cholesterol and reduce other risk factors for coronary heart disease. As foods that are low on the glycemic index (that is, foods that cause the least fluctuation in blood sugar levels), whole grains may enhance insulin sensitivity and lower the risk of type 2 (adult-onset) diabetes, as will be discussed later in the chapter. (*American Journal of Clinical Nutrition,* 1999; 70: 307–308)

As more and more research results are published about whole grains, it becomes clearer that they are valuable for much more than just fiber. It is the *whole grain,* literally the *whole food,* that confers the greatest benefit. The individual components of whole grains—nutrients and phytochemicals working together in powerful ways—help protect against chronic diseases such as some types of cancers, heart disease, and diabetes. It is time to examine the evidence.

Whole Grains and Cancer

A review of existing research published in *Nutrition and Cancer* showed that out of twenty-two studies measuring whole-grain intake and a reduced risk of certain cancers (colorectal, colon, rectal, gastric, oral, pharyngeal, tongue, and esophageal), seventeen showed a significant risk reduction with whole-grain consumption.

Refined grain consumption may boost the risk of stomach cancer. M.C.J.F. Jansen studied the eating habits and risk of diseases among 12,000 middle-aged men from seven countries. The studies showed that men with diets high in refined-grain products also ate relatively little fruit. High fruit consumption was associated with a lower risk of stomach cancer, and consumption of highly refined grain products increased the risk of cancer. (*Nutrition and Cancer*, 1999; 34: 49–55)

Refined-grain consumption also may increase the risk of several other types of cancer. In studies of 2,711 patients in Italy who were hospitalized for various types of cancer, those who consumed the most refined grains (mainly refined flours used in breads and pastas, and white rice) were twice as likely to develop thyroid cancer, compared with people who ate relatively few refined-grain products. Those who ate the most refined grains had a 60 percent higher risk of cancer of the mouth, pharynx, larynx, or esophagus, a 50 percent higher risk of stomach or colon cancer, and a 30 percent higher risk of rectal cancer. (*American Journal of Clinical Nutrition*, 1999; 70: 1107–1110)

A Finnish study found that consumption of whole-grain rye bread significantly improves bowel function and may decrease the risk of colon cancer. Seventeen healthy Finnish men and women, twenty-eight to fifty-one years of age, ate either whole-grain rye bread or refined-wheat bread for four weeks. Fecal output and bowel movement frequency were significantly greater, and the average intestinal time was significantly shorter, for those who ate the whole-grain bread. Additionally, the concentration of some compounds that are thought to be risk markers for cancer were significantly lower in the participants who ate whole-grain rye bread. (*Journal of Nutrition*, Sept 2000; 130: 2215–2221)

Whole Grains and Heart Disease

Whole-grain consumption lowers the risk of heart disease, according to the findings of Yangsoo Jang, M.D., Ph.D., at Yonsei University in Seoul, Korea. Patients with heart disease who ate whole grains and legumes in place of refined grains experienced heart-healthy changes. Their blood glucose levels dropped an average of 24 percent, and insulin levels dropped an average of 14 percent. Both high glucose and high insulin levels are indicators to be heeded as they may be cautionary warnings of heart disease. Vitamin E intake increased an average of 41 percent; and fiber intake, 41 percent. (*Arteriosclerosis, Thrombosis, and Vascular Biology*, Dec 2001)

The American Heart Association, the USDA's *Dietary Guidelines for Americans*, and Healthy People 2010 all recommend that consumers choose a variety of grains, and at least half should be whole grains. Better yet, why not suggest a goal of *all* whole grains?

Whole Grains and Blood Pressure

Whole-grain cereals may benefit individuals with high blood pressure (hypertension). In one study, researchers randomly assigned eighty-six hypertensive patients to eat two whole-grain, oat-based cereals or two refined-grain, wheat-based cereals daily for three months. In the whole-grain group, 73 percent of the patients were able to reduce their antihypertensive medication by half, whereas in the refined-grain group, only 42 percent of patients achieved this result. Furthermore, among those whose medication was not reduced, those eating the whole-grain cereals experienced a more significant drop in systolic pressure than those eating refined cereals. The whole-grain group also experienced a slightly greater drop in diastolic pressure than the refined-grain group, although the amount was regarded as nonsignificant. The whole-grain-cereal group showed a significantly greater reduction in total cholesterol (including both LDL and HDL) and plasma glucose than the refined-grain group. All of these features—improved blood pressure control, reduced need for hypertensive medication, and reduced blood lipid and glucose levels—help reduce the risk of cardiovascular disease. Although all whole grains have some common features, they also have unique properties. For more accurate results, the study should have compared whole-grain, wheat-based cereals with refined wheat-based cereals, or compared whole-grain oatmeal with refined oatmeal. (*Journal of Family Practice*, 2002; 51: 353–359)

Whole Grains and Stroke

Death from stroke is more common in women than in men. Data from a twelve-year Nurses' Health Study at Harvard, conducted with more than 75,000 women, showed that whole-grain consumption lowered the risk of stroke. The average whole-grain intake ranged from as low as 0.13 servings per day, to as high as 2.70 servings per day. Women with a higher whole-grain intake also ate more healthy foods and followed healthier lifestyle practices than women with low whole-grain intake.

Whole Grains and Diabetes

Simin Liu at the Division of Preventive Medicine at Brigham and Women's Hospital in Boston, together with colleagues at Harvard Medical School, examined the data from the Nurses' Health Study discussed above. The data suggested that whole-grain consumption benefits individuals with type 2 diabetes, but refined-grain consumption increases the risk of diabetes. Based on the food-intake analysis, the data showed that the women who ate the most whole grains had a 38 percent lower risk of developing diabetes. This percentage was slightly lower when other factors such as weight, cigarette and alcohol intakes, family history of diabetes, and the use of dietary supplements were included in the analysis. When the researchers compared the relationship between the ratio of refined to whole grains in diabetic risk, they found that women with the highest refined-grain intake and lowest whole-grain intake had a 57 percent greater risk of developing type 2 diabetes. (*American Journal of Public Health,* 2000; 90: 1409–1415)

These findings were followed by another study of the dietary intake of men at risk of type 2 diabetes, with whole-grain intake as a factor. Data were obtained for 42,898 men who participated in the Health Professionals Follow-Up Study. The men had been free of diabetes and cardiovascular disease in 1986. They were monitored for twelve years. Every four years, they were measured by a food-frequency questionnaire. During the follow-up, 1,197 of the participants developed type 2 diabetes. After adjusting for factors such as age, physical activity, cigarette smoking, alcohol intake, vegetable consumption, and energy (calories), the relative risk of type 2 diabetes was 0.58 in subjects who had been eating whole grains in the highest quintile (the portion of a frequency distribution containing one-fifth of the total sample). (*American Journal of Clinical Nutrition,* 2002: 535–540)

Whole Grains and Obesity

According to a study published in the November 2003 issue of the *American Journal of Clinical Nutrition,* women eating high-fiber, whole-grain foods are 50 percent less likely to experience major weight gain over a twelve-year period. And because a high intake of whole-grain foods results in weight control, such a diet also lowers the risk of diabetes.

A study showed that overweight people who can be persuaded to eat whole grains rather than refined ones can manage their blood-sugar concentrations better. This finding corroborates earlier studies and helps to explain why whole grains in the diet lower the risks of type 2 diabetes and heart disease.

Carbohydrates from grains (and other foods) are converted in the body into glucose, a sugar that circulates through the blood until the hormone insulin directs energy-lacking cells to absorb it. Some people develop insulin resistance, a condition in which response to insulin is muted, which forces the body to produce excess insulin to maintain a healthy blood level of glucose. This condition, known as low-insulin sensitivity, increases the risk of type 2 diabetes and heart disease.

Previous research suggested that diets high in refined grains such as white flour and white rice contribute to these diseases. Some data implicate insulin sensitivity as a middle link in the chain of causation.

To test how the intake of whole grain or refined grain affect insulin sensitivity, Mark A. Pereira, lead investigator from the Children's Hospital in Boston, chose eleven overweight or obese subjects between twenty-five and fifty-six years of age who displayed high levels of insulin. They were assigned randomly to consume for six weeks a diet including foods made from either whole or refined grains. The foods included cereal, bread, rice, pastas, muffins, cookies, and snacks. After six weeks on the whole-grain diet, the participants' insulin was 10 percent lower than those on the refined-grain diet. Insulin sensitivity dropped.

Although this was a modest study, with only eleven subjects, Pereira reported that the findings suggest that whole-grain foods would help prevent diabetes. The beneficial effect of whole grains may be due, in part, to their high-fiber content, which slows absorption of carbohydrates and results in a steady delivery of glucose into the bloodstream, with minimal insulin production. Also, the high concentration of minerals in whole grains, such as zinc, copper, and magnesium, plays a role in blood-sugar regulation.

Paul Jacques, D.Sc., M.D., at the USDA's Jean Mayer Human Nutrition Research Center on Aging at Tufts University reviewed data from the Framingham Heart Study of 3,000 middle-aged adults. Jacques found that those who consumed the most whole-grain food had a lower body mass index (BMI), lower waist-to-hips ratio, lower total and LDL cholesterol levels, and improved insulin sensitivity. All of these factors are considered to be markers for a reduced risk of cardiovascular disease and type 2 diabetes. Jacques commented, "The importance of understanding the role of different carbohydrate sources in the development of insulin resistance is becoming ever more critical, because Americans appear to be increasing the intake of dietary carbohydrates." (*American Journal of Clinical Nutrition*, 2002; 76: 390–398)

Insulin resistance, also known as metabolic syndrome, is a condition marked by a combination of abdominal obesity, high triglycerides, low HDL cholesterol, high blood pressure, and poor blood-sugar control. All of these factors increase the risk of developing diabetes and heart disease. A recent study, conducted by Nicola McKeown, a nutritional epidemiologist, and her colleagues at the Human Nutrition Research Center on Aging demonstrated that individuals who consumed at least three whole-grain food servings daily were less apt to develop metabolic syndrome than those eating refined grain products.

Whole Grains and Longevity

Data from a ten-year Iowa Women's Health Study associated the consumption of whole-grain foods with a substantially lower mortality rate. The study, conducted from 1986 to 1996, showed that women aged fifty-five to sixty-nine years had a 15 to 25 percent reduction in death from all causes, including cardiovascular disease and cancer, if their diets included at least one serving daily of whole-grain foods. The lead author of the study, David R. Jacobs, Jr., Ph.D., professor of epidemiology at the University of Minnesota at Minneapolis, reported that the results had important public health implications and urged the general population to increase its whole-grain food intake.

Jacobs, like Joanne L. Slavin, Ph.D., R.D., professor of nutrition at the University of Minnesota at St. Paul, believes that the nutrients in whole grains, including vitamins, minerals, fiber, antioxidants, and phytoestrogens, may act synergistically to fight conditions such as heart disease and cancer. Jacobs reported in the March 1999 issue of the *American Journal of Public Health* that, "The study of individual food components may mask whole grains' total health effect. This reasoning may help explain why interpretation of data from the Harvard Nurses' Health Study appeared to find no association between fiber consumption and a reduced risk of colon cancer."

Whole Grains and Learning

Studies conducted at Tufts University showed that children who eat hot cooked oatmeal perform better on memory tasks than those who eat cold ready-to-eat cereals, or those who eat no breakfast at all. Thirty children aged nine to twelve years were fed breakfast for three weeks, or given no breakfast. More than half of the children who ate the cooked whole-grain cereal performed better than those who ate the cold ready-to-eat cereal on tasks of spatial memory, which is important for mathematical and geographical skills. More than three-fourths of the children who ate the cooked whole-grain cereal performed better than the children who ate no breakfast.

Commenting on the results of this study, Robin Kanarek, Ph.D., professor of psychology and nutrition at Tufts University, reported at the thirty-first annual meet of the Society for Neuroscience held in San Diego, California on November 12, 2001, that "Oatmeal's whole-grain, high-fiber, and protein attributes are believed to be some of the primary factors in increasing spatial memory performance in young children. These nutritional attributes help delay digestion and promote a slower and prolonged release of glucose in the blood system. The improved performance with oatmeal suggests that this process may enhance cognitive performances because the brain is dependent on a constant supply of glucose to satisfy its energy demands."

Acknowledging Whole Grains

In October 2004, General Mills, Inc., announced plans to become the nation's first leading food manufacturer to reformulate all of its Big G breakfast cereals with whole grains. The announcement led David Kessler, M.D., former commissioner of the U.S. Food and Drug Administration (FDA), to commend General Mills' actions. Kessler suggested that "the increased use of whole grains might signal the most comprehensive improvement in the nation's food supply since the government began mandatory fortification of grains in the late 1940s."

Another development was the introduction of a new flour by ConAgra Food Ingredients called Ultragrain White Whole Wheat flour. The new flour is made from a patented process that had been in development for nearly a decade. The flour is 100 percent whole wheat, but the particle size of the grain is reduced to that of refined flour. To consumers accustomed to white flour, Ultragrain White Whole Wheat flour might be more acceptable than the typical whole-wheat flour. However, the new flour has drawbacks. Past studies have shown that coarsely ground flour is more desirable than finely ground flour, in terms of its glycemic effect as well as its effectiveness as a source of dietary fiber. In nanotechnology, smaller particles do not necessarily act in the same way as customary larger-sized particles.

By the late 1990s, there was a preponderance of scientific evidence regarding the values of whole grains and the shortcomings of their refinements. By 1999, the FDA allowed manufacturers of foods containing 51 percent or more of whole-grain ingredients, by weight, to use a health claim on their product labels. (See "Defining a Whole Grain" on page 78.)

Originally, the Food Guide Pyramid devised by the USDA did not specify that grain servings should be chosen from whole grains. The agency took some belated action in harmony with the labeling claim and began to suggest that at least half of grain foods consumed should be whole grains. This recommendation is repeated in the 2005 revised Food Guide Pyramid, accompanied by the number of ounces of grains that should be consumed daily: 8 ounces for men; 6, for women; and 5, for children. This translates to 4 ounces of whole grains for men; 3, for women; and 2.5, for children. How practical are these recommendations?

These actions, although laudatory, are halfway measures. They acknowledge the scientific findings but allow leeway for millers, bakers, and consumers unwilling to make radical dietary changes. To understand the issue, one needs some historical perspective.

The experience in World War II, both in America and England, made government officials leery of a big shift in diet. During wartime, to make the best use of all food resources, both governments mandated that millers use high-extraction rates in flour grindings, to conserve nutrients. As a result, these populations ate mostly whole grains, and despite certain wartime food shortages and curtailments, the people thrived. However, after the war ended, the millers succeeded in pressuring the governments to relax restrictions. The millers returned to their prewar practice of producing refined flours. In recognition of the shortcomings of these products, the United States government made a feeble attempt to improve flour by the enrichment program. Although the program was well intentioned, as described earlier, it is without merit.

There are barriers to whole-grain consumption, as reflected in surveys. Consumers cannot recognize whole-grain foods. They think, erroneously, that all whole-grain foods are dark in color. For example, an oat-based product may not be perceived as a whole-grain product, even though it may be one. Also, not all brown grain products are whole grain. The darkness may be achieved by the addition of caramel coloring to the product.

Other barriers described by consumers are texture, lack of softness, dryness, and unappealing taste of whole-grain products. Other consumers have reported that they would purchase and consume whole-grain products if they were inexpensive and convenient. Americans continue to consume foods made mostly with refined flours. *Currently, whole grains represent only one percent of the total calories consumed by the average American.*

Professor Joanne L. Slavin, mentioned earlier as a prominent researcher of whole grains, challenged food processors to develop whole-grain products that overcome the consumer objections expressed in the surveys. Although the health claim allowed by the FDA was successful in promoting whole grains, it is difficult for processed foods, other than plain whole-grain cereals that require cooking, to meet the health-claim requirements. Bread bakers, unaccustomed to using whole-grain flours, found that they could use up to 25 percent of whole-grain flours, by weight of the flours, but higher amounts of whole-grain ingredients created processing problems. To qualify for the health claims the product must contain at least 51 percent whole-grain ingredients. The bakers claim that pretreating the grains helps, but this increases their costs. Also, the hardness of the whole grains can dull bread

---

DEFINING A WHOLE GRAIN

Numerous surveys show that food technologists, dietitians, and consumers alike are unclear about what constitutes a "whole grain." The Whole Grain Council in Boston, Massachusetts, (a consortium of scientists, chefs, and industry representatives, formed in 2003 by Oldways Preservation Trust, a food-issues think tank) worked with leading grain scientists to formulate a definition. Forthrightly, the Council defined whole grains as foods that contain all essential parts and nutrients of the original grain seed. As a reference, the Council included a list of commonly accepted whole grains. (For more information, see www.wholegrains council.org.)

A more detailed definition of a whole grain was supplied by Professor Dennis T. Gordon, professor of cereal science at North Dakota State University at Fargo in the December 2004 issue of *Food Processing's Wellness Foods* magazine. In describing whole wheat, he said, "It is the kernel with its bran covering, complete aleuron layer, germ, and endosperm." However, Gordon cautioned that "low-extraction flour (72 percent or higher) has no bran and a minimum amount of aleuron layer. Adding wheat bran back to low-extraction flour will not constitute whole wheat."

To a cereal chemist, whole grains include the seeds of grasses, consisting of single kernels (monocotyledons) such as wheat, corn, rice, barley, oats, millet, rye, triticale, teff, wild rice, and others. Whole grains also include pseudo-cereals (dicotyledons) such as amaranth, buckwheat, quinoa, and others. The definition of whole grains would also extend to legumes. The American Association of Cereal Chemists officially endorsed a definition of whole grains to "consist of the intact, ground, cracked, or flaked caryopsis, whose principal anatomical compo-

slicers, which also increases costs. Until consumers clamor for whole-grain products, bakers are reluctant to convert.

Slavin urged the food industry to "think creatively" about how to include whole grains in their products, in view of the scientific evidence that supports the importance of the effort. Slavin also urged the food industry to label whole-grain products clearly so that consumers can identify them readily.

SHOPPING FOR WHOLE-GRAIN BREADS, CRACKERS, AND CEREALS

Even when consumers search for products containing 100 percent whole-grain flour, label reading can be confusing. Many terms are used that do *not*

---

nents—the starchy endosperm, germ, and bran—are present in substantially the same proportions as they exist in the intact caryopsis." Critics suggest that this definition allows too much leeway in determining exactly what "substantially the same proportions" means, and that processors may push this boundary too far.

In 1999, the Food and Drug Administration (FDA) allowed food products that contained 51 percent or more of whole-grain ingredients by weight to include a health claim on the label, as long as the product is low in total fats, saturated fat, and cholesterol. The FDA chose to authorize this whole-grain-food health claim by using dietary fiber as the index for a standard of compositional identity. However, the agency *did not establish a definition of whole grain.* No clear standard of identity for its whole-grain status was defined for any cereal.

The Whole Grain Council feels that consumers need some means of identifying whole-grain products at a glance on packages, without having to read a long list of ingredients. The Council is developing a packaging logo to help shoppers determine the amount of whole grain in a product. It hopes to develop an easily identifiable logo that "will identify three levels of whole-grain goodness . . . three levels will designate products with a half serving of whole grain; a full serving; and . . . products that are 100 percent whole grain."

General Mills submitted a citizen's petition to the FDA requesting new health claims to describe a food product containing at least 8 grams of whole grains per serving as a "good" source of whole grain, and one with 16 grams of whole grains as an "excellent" source. The Whole Grain Council has submitted a petition for a third level that would state "100 percent whole grain."

The FDA will need to respond to these packaging claims and the Whole Grain Council logo.

denote whole grains. For example, "wheat flours," "multigrain," "stone-ground wheat," "unbleached wheat," "enriched wheat," "natural wheat," or "organic wheat" are some of the terms used on food labels of products that do *not* contain 100 percent whole grain. Nor is pumpernickel a whole grain; it consists mainly of white flour, with caramel coloring. Terms such as "7-grain bread," "12-grain bread," and others can be misleading. The grains are not necessarily whole grains, and such breads may contain as little as one-third the fiber content of whole-grain breads.

The label must list on the ingredient panel "whole-wheat flour" or "100 percent whole-wheat flour." "Made with whole-wheat flour" followed by a list of other flours such as "enriched," "fortified," or simply "wheat flour," all denote that the product is less than 100 percent whole grain.

According to Dina Khader, R.D., a nutritional consultant in Mount Kisco, New York, only a small fraction of such products contain high amounts of whole grains. Many actually contain higher amounts of refined grains and lack the fiber-rich bran and the nutrient-rich germ.

If the whole-grain product is made from rice, the label should read "100 percent brown rice"; and if the product is made from corn, "whole corn-meal" or "undegerminated cornmeal" should appear on the label.

Many of the marketed grain products touted as "high in fiber" account for an estimated 95 percent of grains being consumed, noted David J. A. Jenkins, M.D., Ph.D., a clinical nutritionist at the University of Toronto. Jenkins suggested that eating refined-grain products supplemented with wheat bran probably does not offer the health benefits of improved insulin sensitivity, which is offered by whole-grain products. (*Agricultural Research,* Dec 2004)

Whole-Grain Breads

If you shop for whole-grain breads, and read labels carefully, you will make the shocking discovery that few products in supermarkets actually are 100 percent whole grains. Those that are may still be poor choices if they also contain undesirable ingredients and chemical additives.

Better whole-grain bread choices exist in health/natural food stores. However, even in these stores, careful label reading is essential. Many of the breads carried in these stores are not 100 percent whole grain. Ironically, the best choices sometimes come from Europe (especially Germany). Breads such as Hümmlinger are vacuum packaged, double wrapped, and made with all-organic or biodynamic ingredients. Such breads are dense, chewy, and flavorsome. Even one slice gives a good feeling of satiety.

Whole-Grain Crackers

Whole-grain crackers are also difficult to locate. Sometimes they are termed "crisp bread." Unfortunately, most domestically produced crackers, even when made from 100 percent whole-grain flours, often contain objectionable ingredients such as hydrogenated fats and synthetic antioxidants such as BHT and BHA. One satisfactory domestically produced cracker is Ak-Mak, a cracker made from 100 percent stone-ground whole wheat (Ak-Mak Bakeries, 89 Academy Ave., Sanger, CA 93657; 559-264-4145). Some imported crackers are acceptable. Finn Crisp, a Finnish cracker, consists solely of whole rye flour, salt, yeast, and caraway seeds. Some Wasa crackers from Sweden are 100 percent whole-grain products, including Sourdough Rye, Hearty Rye, Fiber Rye, and Light Rye. Read the labels carefully on Wasa crackers. Not all of the products are made from 100 percent whole grains. Ryvita, a cracker made in England, is another whole-grain product, made simply from whole-grain rye, sesame seeds, and salt (The Ryvita Company, Ltd., Old Wareham Road, Poole, Dorset, England BH12 4QW; www.ryvita.com).

Whole-Grain Cereals

Selecting a whole-grain cereal is, again, tricky. Such products are practically nonexistent in supermarkets, despite the dizzying array of costly ready-to-eat dry cereals on shelves. Usually, you can find plain brown rice and plain rolled oats (some instant), but you can find superior counterparts to these cereals sold in bins in health/natural food stores.

At the mention of hot cooked cereal, most people think of oatmeal. If you use oatmeal, try the steel-cut rather than the rolled oats. Sometimes steel-cut oatmeal is known as Irish oatmeal. In the British Isles, it is called porridge. However, oatmeal is but one of a number of whole grains suitable for cereal. Although many people think of using rice with a main meal, or in soups or casseroles, rice can serve as a breakfast cereal, too. There are different varieties of rice available: brown, mahogany, and japonica black, among others.

Rotate whole-grain cereals for variety. Each one has unique qualities. Also, rotation helps to prevent the buildup of allergic reactions that can develop when one eats the same food, repeatedly, for extended periods of time.

Health/natural food stores stock many whole grains suitable for use as cereals, or to be added to soups or stews. Buy them from the bulk bins, whenever possible, for the simplest and least expensive whole grains. Make certain that the stock is fresh and clean. Also whenever possible, obtain whole grains that are organically or biodynamically grown.

In health/natural food stores, you will find some of the following whole grains in bins: amaranth, barley, buckwheat, bulgur (parched wheat), un-degerminated cornmeal, Job's tears, millet, steel-cut oatmeal, quinoa, brown rice and other rices, and teff. These can be cooked whole. Additionally, there are some whole grains in bins that must be cracked before you cook them as cereal: rye and whole-wheat "berries"; kamut and spelt (forerunners of wheat); and triticale (a composite of wheat and rye). You can crack these grains with a mortar and pestle. Or you can use an electric seed grinder, blender, or food processor by "pulsing" briefly; if you continue too long, the product will be flour. Plan to crack the grains just prior to cooking them.

Health/natural food stores also sell many packaged ready-to-eat cereals that are made with whole grains. Such products may seem appealing because of convenience. However, they are poorer choices than simple whole grains that you can cook. To process the grains for the ready-to-eat cereals, the grains are exposed to high heat and pressure to convert them into flakes or puffs, and their nutritional values are reduced drastically. Also, other ingredients added to these products may be undesirable. Such products are high-profit items.

When you arrive home with the whole-grain cereals selected from the bins, transfer the bagged grains to tightly closed glass containers and store them in a dry, cool place. They do not require refrigeration as long as they remain whole and are stored properly. They have a long shelf life.

PREPARING WHOLE GRAINS

A simple rule of thumb for preparing whole grains is to use about twice as much liquid as grain for a cooked whole-grain cereal. For each serving, measure about $1/4$ cup of whole grain and put it in a cooking pot. Add about 1 tablespoon of liquid whey to $1/2$ cup of water, and pour the mixture over the grain. Stir, cover the pot, and allow it to stand overnight at room temperature. In the morning, cook the cereal for ten to twenty minutes, depending on the grain. For example, bulgur and buckwheat cook quickly, whereas millet and steel-cut oats require longer cooking. All of the liquid should be absorbed and the grain should be well cooked.

Note: Whey enhances digestibility of the cereal. You can obtain whey by making yogurt cheese (see "How to Make Yogurt Cheese" on page 147). Store the unused portion of whey in the refrigerator. It will keep for several months. Or, you can buy dried whey in a health/natural food store and reconstitute it in water. A heaping tablespoon of whey dissolved in $1/2$ cup of water is a good proportion.

Obviously, it is best to use grains whole, not in a refined state. As indicated, many grains can be used whole, as cereals, in soups, stews, and casseroles, or as starch dishes such as brown rice. Grains that require cracking, such as rye and wheat berries, should be cracked roughly. Grains milled into flour also should be ground coarsely rather than finely to maintain the integrity of the grains' physical properties. This brings us to a consideration of the glycemic index.

Whole Grains and the Glycemic Index

The glycemic index (GI) was devised in the early 1970s by Gerald Reaven, M.D., an endocrinologist, and his colleagues at Stanford Medical School in California. The group began to investigate the rates at which different starches break down in the body. The researchers learned that starches release glucose at very different rates. Baked potato and bread release glucose quickly, whereas cooked corn and rice release glucose more slowly. The researchers found that the gut digests rice at different rates, depending on the degree of milling of the grain. This finding demonstrated the importance of the physical properties of a food.

Nutritionists promptly incorporated these findings about the GI values of individual foods into their dietary recommendations for diabetics. They advised diabetic patients who needed to control their blood sugar level to consume less of processed foods.

However, the GI findings were important, as well, for nondiabetics who make adequate amounts of insulin yet have difficulty in using the hormone. In these people, certain tissues, especially in muscle and fat, cannot absorb glucose from blood unless it is assisted by insulin. In this condition, known as insulin resistance, normal concentrations of insulin are insufficient, and the body begins to compensate by producing increasingly larger amounts of insulin. The more insulin resistant a person becomes, the more insulin the person makes. Eventually, this process can lead to type 2 diabetes. Reaven contended that for a growing number of Americans with insulin resistance, carbohydrate-rich diets are hazardous.

A decade after Reaven and his colleagues presented their findings, studies with the GI were furthered by clinical nutritionist David J. A. Jenkins. Jenkins, too, was concerned that certain carbohydrates might be hazardous to individuals who are insulin resistant. To evaluate the risks, Jenkins investigated the breakdown rates of carbohydrate foods. Jenkins and his colleagues fed a battery of foods to healthy individuals and ranked the foods' GI on a 100-point scale. Pure glucose rated at the top at 100. The higher the

GI value of a food, the more rapidly the carbohydrates convert into blood sugar. Thus, the lower the food measures on the GI, the better it is, in terms of beneficial slower conversion of carbohydrates into blood sugar.

After Jenkins's team measured a range of foods for their GI values, they had volunteers eat diets with a low or high rating. The diets based on low GI carbohydrates resulted in many health benefits. However, it was found that the quantity and quality of a food's fiber was critical to its GI status. It was difficult to ascertain whether the benefits could be attributed simply to the food intake low in GIs, to fibers in the foods, or to both. GI status and fiber seem to be intertwined. Fiber in the carbohydrate foods can slow the digestion, but *only if the fiber remains as an intact part of the original food.*

Studies conducted by Jennie Brand-Miller, Ph.D., at the University of Sydney, Australia, showed that whole grains have GIs of about 50. However, when the grains are milled and their fibers crushed and separated from the rest of the grain, the flours—both whole-grain and refined ones—made into breads, raise their levels in GI measures to about 70. In her book *The Glucose Revolution* (Marlowe & Co., 1999), Brand-Miller observed, "Fiber and GI are intimately mixed up in a way that most people don't understand."

In general, most refined starchy foods eaten by Americans have high GI values, whereas nonstarchy vegetables, fruits, and legumes tend to have low GI values. To some extent, the addition of protein and fat lowers the GI values of individual foods, but does not change their levels on the GI. In recent years, the GI totals and the glycemic load of the average American diet have risen because of increased carbohydrate consumption and changes that have occurred in food processing.

In part, official dietary recommendations are to blame. The original USDA Food Guide Pyramid, recommending the inordinate number of six to twelve servings daily of cereal-grain foods, failed to specify what grains they were to be. Americans took this advice as an endorsement for all manner of pastas, and baked goods such as cakes, pies, muffins, and cookies. Six to twelve servings of such foods displace more nutritious ones from the diet. Nor did the original Food Guide Pyramid make any distinction between whole-grain flours and refined ones. Only as an afterthought a decade later did the USDA issue the weak recommendation that half of the cereal-grain intake should be from whole grains. The 2005 revised Food Guide Pyramid repeats the same recommendation.

Selections from Jenkins's list of GI values demonstrate that the greater the refinement of flour, the higher the GI value. Jenkins found that instant rice had a GI value of 91; white rice, 72; and brown rice, 66. The GI value for white bread was 69; rye bread, 66. The packaged ready-to-eat cereals showed cornflakes at 80; Swiss muesli, 66; All-Bran, 51; and oatmeal, 49. (Measurements by other researchers vary slightly from Jenkins's measures, but in general, the pattern is consistent.)

Remember that the GI is a scale of 1 to 100 that rates how quickly specific foods raise blood sugar. The GI works only as a measure of individual foods. The addition of other foods, especially proteins and fats, slows down the digestive process and prevents the blood sugar from spiking and crashing.

Acrylamide and Starchy Foods

The benefit of using whole grains as a cooked cereal, or in moist cooking such as simmering or stewing, has been given additional support recently from an unsuspected problem that has emerged: acrylamide.

Acrylamide, commercially produced since 1954, is a substance widely used in the production of plastic polymers, dyes, and adhesives. It is also used as a flocculant (a substance that forms masses of waste so that it can be reused) for sewage and waste treatment, and for soil conditioning and ore processing. What does acrylamide have to do with foods, and especially starchy ones?

The presence of acrylamide in food was a chance discovery. In 1997, researchers at Stockholm University in Sweden were testing tunnel workers exposed to large quantities of acrylamide from a water sealant. After finding high levels of acrylamide both in these workers and in workers who had not been exposed to the sealant, the researchers conducted further tests and concluded that the source of the substance came from the workers' diets. Acrylamide was found in commonly used cooked starchy staple foods, especially ones cooked at high temperatures. Acrylamide was found in potato chips and French fries. However, of importance to our discussion of grain foods, acrylamide was also found, at lower levels, in baked goods such as cookies, processed cereals, and breads. Levels of acrylamide varied between brands. Acrylamide was found in the tested foods at levels that were hundreds of times higher than the maximal level of 0.5 micrograms (mcg) per liter (l) considered safe for drinking water by the World Health Organization (WHO) and the U.S. Environmental Protection Agency (EPA). The higher the cooking temperature and the longer the cooking time, the more acrylamide was detected.

This finding was worrisome to public health officials. Workers who manufacture acrylamide are cautioned that the substance is highly toxic and irritating. It can be absorbed through unbroken skin. Acrylamide is classified as a human neurotoxin and can cause nervous system paralysis. Also, it is classified as an acknowledged carcinogen in rats and a probable carcinogen in humans. It is classified, too, as a genotoxicant, which is a substance that can mutate and damage genetic material. Acrylamide, as a genotoxicant, has been shown to lead to several different types of cancer formations in rats: breast and uterine cancers, tumors of the adrenal glands, and tumors in the internal lining of the scrotum. In animal studies, acrylamide tends to attack the thyroid gland, female mammary gland, male testes, and the mouth.

As a result of the Swedish findings, on April 24, 2002, Sweden's National Food Administration announced that acrylamide may be formed in high concentrations when carbohydrate-rich foods are heated at high levels. Follow-up studies, conducted in Norway, Switzerland, the United Kingdom, Canada, and the United States, with hundreds of food samples, confirmed the Swedish findings. The findings were sensational.

On June 25, 2002, WHO convened a panel of twenty-three food scientists in Geneva to discuss the scientific evidence and to plan additional research. Dr. Dieter Arnold from the Federal Institute of Health Protection of Consumers and Veterinary Medicine in Germany, who chaired the panel, reported that "current limited knowledge does not allow us to answer all the questions which have been asked by consumers, regulators, and other interested parties." However, the panel judged acrylamide formation in food to be "a serious problem." Dr. Arnold stated frankly, "It is the first time we are dealing with substances that are potentially carcinogenic in human staple foods."

Jorgen Schlundt, WHO's Coordinator of Food Safety Research, reported that WHO estimated the total intake of acrylamide from the average Western diet of food and water, and from other sources such as cosmetics and cigarette smoke, to be about 70 mcg daily for an adult. This is significantly below the level that is known to cause nerve damage in laboratory animals, but far higher than the maximal level of 0.5 mcg/l considered safe for drinking water.

However, the true risk is difficult to evaluate. Other carcinogens in foods have similar potency, such as the polycyclic aromatic hydrocarbons (PAHs) that also form when food is heated to high levels in grilling and frying. WHO estimates that acrylamide exposure from the average Western diet is likely to be higher than PAH exposure. *Acrylamide concentrations in affected foods is estimated to be 10 to 1,000 times higher than PAH concentrations.* To date, information is nonexistent about an additive or potentially synergistic effect of PAHs combined with acrylamide. Yet, both compounds commonly are present in the same meal.

After Sweden issued its reports, the Food Standards Agency—the food watchdog of the United Kingdom—began to test food products. The agency found that some products had acrylamide levels 1,280 times higher than international safety limits. Unlike the FDA's policy, the British agency divulged brand names. Kellogg's Rice Krispies, the ready-to-eat cereal, was found to have 110 parts per billion (ppb) of acrylamide. Exceedingly high amounts of acrylamide were found in Walkers Crisps (potato chips) at 1,270 ppb acrylamide, and Pringles, another potato chip, which is familiar to Americans, at 1,400 ppb acrylamide.

Since the identification of acrylamide in starchy staples, scientists in England, Switzerland, Canada, and the United States, working independently of one another, uncovered similar evidence. They found that acrylamide can form in these foods when they are cooked at high temperatures, and especially when they are fried, due to asparagine. This amino acid present in foods, when heated, can combine with reducing sugars (a general term for certain sugars such as glucose, dextrose, levulose, and others that are oxidized readily by alkaline copper sulfate) that are also present in the foods. The combination of asparagine and glucose produces the "Maillard reaction," a development well-known to food scientists. The Maillard reaction is responsible for producing the brownness and agreeable flavor in bread crusts, crackers, and other baked goods.

For years, food technologists have known that the longer bread is baked and the greater its degree of brownness in the crust, the greater the nutritional losses. The newer knowledge is that along with the brownness and crispness comes the additional feature of acrylamide formation.

Scientists noted that the chemical structure of asparagine looks suspiciously like that of acrylamide. Two different teams, one from England and another from Switzerland, investigated. The English group was led by Professor Donald S. Mottram of the University of Reading and Professor Bronek L. Wedzicha of the University of Leeds. Both specialize in food chemistry. The Swiss group was led by Richard H. Stadler of the Nestlé Research Center in Switzerland. Both groups came to similar conclusions. Heating asparagine and glucose to a high temperature produces a significant amount of acrylamide. (*Nature*, 3 Oct 2002; 419: 448–449) Additional studies done by scientists in the United States and in Canada showed similar results.

Different cooking temperatures and cooking times might account for the variability of acrylamide levels found in foods. However, other factors could include the amount of free asparagine, meaning the amount of asparagine that is not bound to another substance, and the availability of sugars in food. Commonly used staples such as grains (wheat or rye) and potatoes contain high levels of free asparagine, and they are rich in carbohydrates.

The FDA presented its acrylamide action plan: to assess human dietary exposures, to gather information about acrylamide's toxicology, and to develop techniques to reduce its formation in foods. The agency began to analyze numerous food products, using a technique that the agency developed. To date, the agency has tested more than 300 food products and plans to test about 1,500 more samples. Based on the findings, more products may be added.

Meanwhile, you as a consumer can protect yourself. Follow the recommendations made both by the Food and Agricultural Organization (FAO) and WHO: do not cook food excessively or at too high a temperature. Although this advice is good, it needs to be extended further. Remember that moist heat, achieved by simmering, poaching, and steaming, is preferable to dry heat that uses long roasting and high heat. Gentle sautéing is preferable to deep-fat frying. Use grilled foods infrequently, if at all. Avoid heavily charred foods. Discard burnt fats, overheated smoked oils, and *beurre noire* (purposely blackened butter). Scrape lightly burnt toast and discard heavily burnt toast. Avoid deep-fried breads, French fries, and potato chips.

Many of the starch products that have been found to contain acrylamide also are low in nutrients. Ready-to-eat cereals are inferior to cooked whole-grain cereals. French fries and potato chips are inferior to baked or boiled potatoes. By choosing foods free of acrylamide, you achieve safety and better nutrition, too.

Grains Are Not for Everyone

Some people are gluten sensitive. Gluten is one of the proteins contained in some grains. Gliadin and glutenin are other proteins that may be involved, too, but gluten is the one usually mentioned. Wheat and rye contain the most gluten; oats and barley contain lesser amounts; spelt and kamut (forerunners of wheat) and triticale (a hybrid of wheat and rye) also contain gluten. Unfortunately, even though all of these gluten-containing whole grains are nutritious, gluten-intolerant individuals must avoid them totally.

The cause of gluten intolerance is a matter of conjecture. One theory is that the condition is due to an intestinal enzyme deficiency, an inborn metabolic error. Lack of the enzyme leads to an incomplete breakdown of gluten, resulting in an accumulation of toxic peptides in the gastrointestinal lumen (cavity). Normally, the enzyme would break down and detoxify the gluten before it could damage the intestinal villi (numerous threadlike projections covering the mucous membrane lining the small intestine and involved in fluid and nutrient absorption).

Another theory is that gluten intolerance is due to the presence of abnormal gluten-binding sites on the epithelial cells in the intestinal tract. This results in gluten binding to these cells and their destruction.

Yet another theory is that gluten intolerance is due to an immunologic defect, which somehow inactivates many of the gastrointestinal epithelial cells.

Also, it has been suggested that an intestinal viral infection may play a role. An encounter of the immune system with an antigen produced during an intestinal viral infection may be important in the development of gluten intolerance.

Although the cause of gluten intolerance may be unclear, the manifestation of the condition is real. It can appear at any age and is essentially similar for all age groups. Gluten intolerance is not outgrown. A lifetime of *total* avoidance of gluten-containing grains is vital.

Gluten intolerance is not a new disease. Only its designation is new. Celiac disease, its common name, has been recognized for about 2,000 years. As early as the second century A.D., Greek physicians noted that diet played a significant role in the well-being of *koiliakos* sufferers. They observed that bread was rarely suitable to strengthen *koiliakos* children.

In India, intestinal diseases, including what we assume to be sprue and other celiac diseases, were described in the medical literature in Sanskrit, as early as 1500 B.C. The first known European treatise on celiac disease dates from the second century A.D. Its author, Aretaeus, coined the term "coeliac," from the Greek word for "belly" to describe the abdominal distension experienced by sufferers of this condition. In 1669, the Dutch physician Vincent Katelaer described "Stomatitis Aphthous" in his treatise on "spruw." He noted numerous small ulcers in the intestines as well as in the mouths of sufferers of debilitating diarrhea.

Later, many medical references designated celiac disease as a childhood illness, and sprue or nontropical sprue as an adulthood illness. All of these terms designate gluten intolerance.

Individuals who are gluten intolerant must avoid gluten because this grain protein alters the cellular lining of the small intestine. The villi are flattened or even absent. Under these conditions, gluten in contact with the small intestine can lead to malabsorption of many nutrients. Malabsorption can contribute to many health problems, including high blood pressure, heart irregularities, and conditions related to low serum calcium. If malabsorption is undiagnosed, misdiagnosed, or diagnosed properly but ignored, it can lead to neurological disorders, intestinal ulceration, and even intestinal cancer.

Symptoms of gluten intolerance reflect indigestion. There may be abdominal distension and irritable bowel. Stools may be pale, greasy, bulky, and malodorous. These symptoms may be accompanied by diarrhea, headache, nausea, and vomiting. Appetite may be poor. Drowsiness may follow meals. There may be anemia, weight loss, and skin pallor. There may be muscle cramps and spasms, bone or joint pains, and in times of stress, a flare-up of these symptoms. Although these various symptoms may be attributed to numerous causes, gluten intolerance may be overlooked.

In addition to avoiding gluten-containing whole grains, reading labels is essential to avoid gluten used in different ways. Several decades ago, chemically altered starch, known as modified food starch (or simply food starch) was introduced into food manufacturing to serve technical needs. Such starch now appears in virtually all processed foods, and the specific grain from which it is derived is unnamed. Commonly, starches, emulsifiers, and stabilizers are made from wheat.

The use of gluten has been extended to many food products that formerly were free of grain constituents. Among many applications, wheat gluten is used as a formulation aid, binder, filler, bulking agent, shaper, and aid in making tablets. Gluten can inhibit cooking losses, prevent shrinkage from moisture losses, emulsify fat and other substances, bind juices in food products, and improve the texture of many foods. Gluten may be added to formulated meat and poultry products, such as restructured steaks, meat rolls, sausage products (including beef, pork, and fish), and to textured protein meat extenders and meat analogs. Dried distillers' grain flour may be used as an ingredient in canned meat-based foods. Gluten is added to imitation cheeses to improve their stretchability, and to foods to prevent them from becoming mushy when they are held for long periods on steam tables in restaurants. Gluten is used as a substrate for hydrolysis in the manufacturing of those two ubiquitous flavor enhancers: monosodium glutamate (MSG) and vegetable protein hydrolysate, also known as hydrolyzed vegetable protein (HVP). Malt, used mainly as a flavoring and coloring agent, can be a hidden source of gluten. Most ready-to-eat breakfast cereals, including those from grains not containing gluten, contain malt or malt extract. Although gluten is not contained in wheat germ, it may contaminate it. One major wheat-germ processor reported that because the germ is separated from the wheat kernel through mechanical means, it is possible that some element in the germ could have a small amount of gluten.

Obviously, a gluten-intolerant individual is served best by selecting basic whole foods and avoiding processed ones. Fortunately, there are whole grains that do not contain gluten. Amaranth, buckwheat (not a true grain), undegerminated cornmeal, Job's tears, millet, quinoa, various rices, and teff are whole grains that may be tolerated by individuals who are sensitive to gluten. None of these grains contain gluten.

There are other individuals who also seem to respond unfavorably to whole grains, according to James Braly, M.D., and Ron Hoggan, coauthors of *Dangerous Grains* (Avery Publishing Group, 2002). They relate gluten, gliadin, and glutenin to more than 200 chronic health problems and diseases that can be experienced in individuals with non-celiac gluten sensitivity. They claim that health professionals fail to differentiate between celiac disease and non-celiac gluten sensitivity, and may give unsatisfactory medical advice to the latter group. Positive test results indicating non-celiac gluten sensitivity may be dismissed, assuming that such results are nonspecific. Such patients may not be encouraged to follow a strict non-gluten diet. More commonly, their immune reactions to gluten may not even be mentioned, or the reactions may be dismissed as irrelevant.

Some of the health problems that may have gluten sensitivity as a factor include autoimmune diseases, osteoporosis, brain disorders, intestinal diseases and disorders, and cancers. People with conditions such as multiple sclerosis, rheumatoid arthritis, Sjögren's syndrome, dermatitis herpetiformis, regional enteritis, diabetes, infertility, autism, and schizophrenia have experienced some degree of amelioration by excluding gluten-containing grains from their diet.

Why is gluten intolerance experienced? The domestication of cereal grains is relatively recent in the history of humankind. Such cereal grains have been in existence for some 10,000 years, a brief span of time. Their introduction challenged the human metabolic system by altering its nutritional composition. Humans shifted from their traditional role as food gatherers (hunting and gathering) to a new role as food producers (agriculture). This shift wrought revolutionary dietary changes that, for a significant number of persons, may have proved too drastic for rapid adaptation to the digestive tract. However, for the many who have adapted, whole grains are nutritious whole foods that contribute to a mixed diet.

Chapter 4

Nutrient-Dense Nuts and Seeds

Once stigmatized as a food to be avoided,
experts are now praising health benefits of eating nuts.
—Sylvia Rector, *Journal Star*, Peoria, Illinois, December 5, 2001

Seeds: The Germs of Life

—Theme for *New York's Food & Life Sciences Conference*, 1981
(Cornell University, Ithaca, New York)

Nuts and seeds have been part of the human diet from the time of the hunter-gatherers. Very recently, evidence of the use of these foods was unearthed from Gesher Benot Ya'aqov, a site in Jerusalem being studied by archaeologists from Hebrew University. Approximately 780,000 years ago at Gesher Benot Ya'aqov, which is along a shoreline in what is now northern Israel, humans ate a varied diet that included almonds, pistachios, and other hard-shelled nuts, according to Naama Goren-Inbar and her colleagues. The researchers were able to find seeds and other remains from seven species of nuts. Four of the species—acorn, almond, pistachio, and water chestnut—have hard outer shells that must be cracked open before eating. The researchers unearthed fifty-four stone implements bearing surface depressions produced by some type of repetitive pounding. The size, shape, and texture of the markings closely resemble the pitting on nut-cracking stones used by modern hunter-gatherers, as well as chimpanzees. According to the scientists, the small nut-cracking stones served as hammers; the larger ones, as anvils.

Goren-Inbar suggests that females at Gesher Benot Ya'aqov probably took care of gathering the nuts and preparing them for eating, while males probably assumed responsibility for hunting and butchery activities, for which much fossil evidence exists. The fat- and protein-rich nuts contributed nutrition to their mixed diet. (*Proceedings of the National Academy of Sciences,* 19 Feb 2002)

Botanically, a nut is a fruit containing a single seed with a hard shell and a tough fruit layer. As commonly viewed, a nut is simply an edible kernel in a hard shell. Nuts are from many diverse botanical families. For example, the hazelnut (also known as filbert) is from the birch family. The almond is from the rose family and is related to the plum, peach, and apricot.

Formerly, nuts were relegated to a lowly role as garnishes. Worse yet, they were shunned or restricted because of their high-fat content. This view was prevalent, especially during the recent low-fat craze.

Finally, nuts have been recognized for their true worth. They are nutrient-dense whole foods that offer many health benefits and should be used in the daily diet. Yet, Americans consume a low volume of nuts. In 1991, the total annual consumption of shelled nuts was only 2.2 pounds per person; in 1992, the same; in 1993 and 1994, 2.3 pounds; then it dipped to 1.9 pounds in 1995 and 1996, probably due to the low-fat craze; 2.1 pounds in 1997; 2.2 pounds in 1998; and a slight rise to 2.5 pounds in 1990 and 2000, probably due to publicity about the health benefits of nuts.

NUTRIENTS IN NUTS

All tree nuts contain similar nutrients, but each type of nut has its own unique nutritional profile. The protein quality score, a measurement of protein quality in food, for most nuts ranges from 46 to 61 percent. Lysine and threonine are the limiting amino acids, that is, the amino acids that limit the protein's value to the diet. Pistachios come close to a 100 percent score but fall short for lysine (97 percent) and threonine (96 percent). For a discussion of the topic of limiting amino acids, see Chapter 5 on protein foods.

Nuts supply arginine, a nonessential amino acid that is a precursor for nitric oxide. Nitric acid may play beneficial roles in the body, including a reduction of cardiovascular disease risk.

Nuts contain 46 to 76 percent total fat, much of which is unsaturated. Macadamia nuts have the highest percentage of saturated fatty acids (SFAs) at 12 percent and monounsaturated fatty acids (MUFAs) at 59 percent. Hazelnuts, pecans, and almonds have MUFAs in a range of 34 to 46 percent. Walnuts have the highest amount of polyunsaturated fatty acids (PUFAs) at 47 percent and the lowest amount of MUFAs at 9 percent. The walnut is the only nut with a significant amount of omega-3 fatty acids (9 percent). This valuable fatty acid, found in fish oils, is rarely found in plant sources. One ounce of walnuts meets the dietary recommendations of the Food and Nutrition Board of the National Academies' Institute of Medicine for daily intake of omega-3 fatty acids.

In a comparison of the nutritive values of different nuts, the USDA estimates that a one-ounce serving of given nuts provides the following:

Nut	Protein (g)	Carbs (g)	Total Fat (g)	SFA (g)	PUFA (g)	Fiber (g)	Calories (g)
Almond	5.7	6.0	15.0	2.0	3.0	3.1	167
Cashew	4.4	9.0	13.0	3.0	2.0	1.5	163
Macadamia	2.4	4.0	21.0	3.0	1.0	NA	199
Pecan	2.2	5.0	19.0	2.0	5.0	1.8	190
Pistachio	5.9	5.0	14.0	2.0	2.0	3.1	160
Walnut	4.1	5.0	18.0	2.0	12.0	1.4	182

Source: Adapted from *USDA Agricultural Handbook,* November 1975.

In addition to their valuable proteins, fats, and fiber, nuts are sources of vitamin B_6 (pyridoxine), folic acid, magnesium, iron, zinc, copper, phosphorus, and potassium. Nuts are a good source of vitamin E, which has antioxidant properties.

Nuts contain no cholesterol and actually may help to reduce or control cholesterol levels, as will be demonstrated in a later discussion. Because of the MUFAs and PUFAs in nuts, they help reduce unfavorable low-density lipoprotein (LDL) cholesterol levels while maintaining high levels of favorable high-density lipoprotein (HDL) cholesterol. Some nuts contain as many as eight different forms of sterols (substances closely related to cholesterol, which also help moderate cholesterol levels).

Perhaps the most exciting findings of all are those from recent investigations of the numerous phytochemicals in nuts. These include carotenoids, flavonoids, indoles, and phenols such as rhamnetin, quercetin, kaempherol aglycones, phenylpropenoids, and benzoic acid derivatives.

NUTS AND HEALTH

The nutrients and phytochemicals in nuts appear to offer many health benefits, including reduced risk of cardiovascular diseases, cancer, and obesity.

Nuts and Cardiovascular Diseases

During the mid-1970s, a team of epidemiologists at Loma Linda University in California asked some 351,000 Seventh-Day Adventists in California to estimate how frequently they ate foods from a submitted list of sixty-five. The participants were over twenty-four years of age. In addition to the questions about foods, there were lifestyle questions. Most Adventists use very little alcohol, caffeinated beverages, or meat. The findings were equivocal regarding the importance of the food list, in view of the confounding factors of lifestyle that also would contribute to good health.

In 1992, a team of researchers led by Gary E. Fraser, M.D., Ph.D., professor of epidemiology at Loma Linda, decided to review the list of foods to learn if any were related to good health. One food stood out: nuts. To a lesser extent, whole-wheat bread was another factor. However, the finding about nuts proved to initiate a turnabout in attitudes regarding fat. Adventists, who consume fat from nuts, live longer than other Americans and experience far fewer heart attacks. This fact challenged the conventional wisdom that fats are associated with cardiovascular diseases. Instead of being a negative factor, fat consumption became a positive one.

Several other large epidemiological studies support the findings of the Loma Linda studies. One is the Nurses' Health Study, conducted with 86,000 women from 1980 to 1990. During that period, there were 1,255 fatal or nonfatal heart attacks experienced by some participants. When the data were analyzed, it was found that of 4,000 women in the group who ate a weekly diet that exceeded 5 ounces a day of all kinds of nuts, only 44 had experienced heart attacks. Of 52,000 women in the group who ate nuts one to four times weekly, there were 555 heart attacks. Of 30,000 women in the group who rarely or never ate nuts, there were 669 heart attacks.

Commenting on these findings, Alice Lichtenstein, D.Sc., a biochemist at the USDA's Jean Mayer Human Nutrition Research Center on Aging at Tufts University said that the new study was valid and important, but "people who tend to eat nuts may be those whose lifestyles are healthier in general." This observation is similar to the earlier one regarding the Adventists. (*NY Times*, 17 Nov 1998, p. D10)

However, Frank B. Hu, Ph.D., of the Harvard School of Public Health and his coworkers, who had analyzed the data, concluded that "an important message from a study like this is that simple lifestyle changes, like eating at least five ounces of nuts each week may help combat heart disease, the leading killer in American women." (*British Medical Journal*, 14 Nov 1998)

In the Nurses' Health Study, among nonsmoking teetotalers who ate nuts, the benefits were even more dramatic. These women experienced only half as much heart disease as the women who rarely ate nuts. (For an analysis of the data from the Nurses' Health Study, see the *British Medical Journal*, 14 Nov 1998: 1341–1345.)

In a study of the effects of nuts (walnuts) on serum lipid levels and blood pressure in normal men, Joan Sabaté, M.D., Ph.D., professor of nutrition and chair of the Department of Nutrition, School of Public Health, at Loma Linda University, reported, "People who ate nuts often—five or more times a week—were half as likely to have a heart attack or die of heart disease as people who rarely or never ate them. Eating nuts just one to four times a week cut the heart risk by a quarter." (*New England Journal of Medicine*, 4 Mar 1993)

Even when the Loma Linda team looked at the data about vegetarian Adventists, those who ate nuts were healthier. "It didn't matter if people were slim or fat, young or old, active or sitting all the time," reported Sabaté and coworkers in the Adventist Health Study. Nuts reduced cardiovascular risks. (*Archives of Internal Medicine*, 1992; 152: 1416-1424)

In one of Sabaté's studies, forty-nine men and women, averaging fifty-six years of age, who had high cholesterol levels, volunteered to eat a diet in which about 35 percent of the energy (calories) was provided by walnuts. The diet was similar to the Mediterranean diet but with walnuts replacing some of the calories from olive oil. Basically, the Mediterranean diet consists of many fruits and vegetables, fish, some wine, and a high level of olive oil. Many of the people on the Mediterranean diet have very low levels of heart disease and cancer, despite the high level of fat in the diet. Incorporating the walnuts into the diet lowered participants' total cholesterol levels by an average of 4.1 percent, and LDL levels by 5.9 percent.

Sabaté said, "We served the whole nut because we were interested in the effect of whole foods served as commonly consumed. The main reason for the cholesterol reduction was the nature of the fat. Walnuts are high in polyunsaturated fat that contains alpha-linolenic acid, which is a precursor of the omega-3 fatty acids found in fish oil. The decrease in cholesterol was even greater than predicted because of other components that may contribute, like fiber and protein." (*Science News*, 13 Mar 1993)

The Physicians' Health Study, a companion to the Nurses' Health Study, also suggests that frequent nut consumption may provide similar heart benefits to men. The study was led by Christine Albert, M.D., an instructor at Harvard Medical School, and funded by the National Institutes of Health (NIH). Albert reported that alpha-linolenic acid may be the factor in the heart-healthy aspect of nuts. This fat is thought to prevent ventricular fibril-lations, a heart disturbance that can lead to sudden death.

The Iowa Women's Health Study, published in the *New England Journal of Medicine* in 1996, provided further support. Results of the study with 34,000 Iowan women showed that those who ate nuts more often than twice weekly reduced their risk of heart problems by 60 percent. They reduced their death rate from cardiovascular disease by 40 percent.

Similar findings were observed in a study led by Gene A. Spiller, Ph.D., D.Sc., C.N.C., director of the Health Research and Studies Center in Los Altos, California, and the Sphera Foundation. A group of twenty-six men and women with high cholesterol ate a few handfuls of almonds daily, in addition to their customary diet. Although the nuts added some fat calories, which rose from 30 to 37 percent, on average, their blood LDL cholesterol levels fell 23 points, while their HDL levels remained constant.

As early as 1980, in a comparison of diets from seven countries, and their heart risk levels, the Mediterranean diet had been declared the most healthful. The Mediterranean diet is higher in fats than the recommended diet in America: 37 percent compared to a maximum of 30 percent. Most of the fat in the Mediterranean diet comes from olive oil. However, Spiller noted that many Mediterranean recipes include almonds. Spiller was intrigued to find out whether almonds, in addition to olive oil, played a role in heart health. Spiller worked along with other researchers from the Universities of Verona, Italy, and Toronto, Canada, to learn what contributions almonds made to the diet. The researchers found that by substituting almonds and almond oil for other fats in the diet for nine weeks, they could lower total and LDL cholesterol.

In a five-week study, the same team compared the effects of almonds, olive oil, or saturated fats in the diet. Saturated fats are abundant in foods from animal sources and from certain plant foods such as coconut and palm oils. They chose forty-five participants who had moderately high cholesterol levels—typically 250 milligrams per deciliter of blood (mg/dl).

During the first week of the trial, the participants were taught to select foods that would comprise a high-fiber, low-saturated-fat meal. The follow-ing week participants were assigned randomly to a diet rich in almonds, olive oil, or saturated fats. The researchers supplied some food daily to the participants. It consisted of about 630 calories, of which about 450 calories were comprised of one of the fat sources. The remainder of the food con-sisted of a mixture of the same healthful offerings given to all groups. The participants supplemented these foods with additional ones that met the study's guidelines for high-fiber, low-saturated-fat meals.

Compared with what the volunteers had been eating during the first week, the new diets increased their caloric intake from fat by 2 to 8 percent. This amounted to 35 percent of calories in the group using saturated fats, and 39 percent of calories in the group using monounsaturated fats (either olive oil or almonds).

After four weeks on the diet, the participants in both of the monounsaturated fat groups showed a drop in total cholesterol levels. Those eating almonds experienced about an 11 percent drop; those eating olive oil, a 4 percent decline. In the group eating the saturated fats, the cholesterol level rose 5 percent. The three diets showed comparable changes in LDL cholesterol levels. The levels fell 17 percent in people eating the diet with almonds and 4 percent in the diet with olive oil. In the diet with saturated fats, the LDL level rose 2 percent.

The amounts of monounsaturated fats are comparable in almonds and olive oil. Why did the almond-consuming group experience greater benefits of changed blood lipid levels than the olive-oil group? Investigations by Paul A. Davis, associate research nutritionist in the department of nutrition, College of Agriculture and Environmental Sciences at the University of California at Davis, may have provided the answer to this question. Davis suggested that the difference may be due to whether the source is from a whole food (almonds, in this case) or a fractionated food (extracted oil, in this case).

According to Davis, some people move the fat that they eat into their blood a little faster than average, and move the fat out of their blood much more slowly than average. Having consumed fat circulate longer in the blood places such individuals at a much higher risk of heart disease than those whose blood circulates fat faster.

Davis investigated whether the source of the fat might be another factor affecting fat-circulation patterns and heart risks. He compared how the body handles equal amounts of fat delivered as whole almonds or almond oil. He found that the timing for absorbing and utilizing almond oil was similar to that of other oils. However, when the almond was consumed as a nut (in a meal, adjusted so that all nutrients and fiber were kept equal to those in meals containing liquid oils), the oil from the nut entered an individual's bloodstream more slowly. It peaked about an hour after consumption and was flushed out rapidly.

As a result of this finding, Davis concluded, "If you eat whole nuts, you deliver fat in a different manner than if you have oils by themselves or as part of [prepared] foods." He added, "It's as if these nuts were time-released pills," slowly releasing their fat in a healthful way. Because all nuts have similar oil-encapsulating structures, "there shouldn't be much difference between a pecan, an almond, or a walnut in terms of its delivery of fat." If Davis is correct, it might explain why the addition of walnuts, which are rather low in monounsaturated fats, nevertheless have been associated with substantial heart benefits, such as a reduced risk of heart attack. (*Science News*, 21 Nov 1998: 329)

Wanda Morgan, Ph.D., associate professor of human nutrition and food science at New Mexico State University in Las Cruces, had participants in a study use self-selected diets. The diets were supplemented with 68 grams of pecans every day. The control group also used a self-selected diet but refrained from eating nuts. By the end of eight weeks, the pecan eaters lowered their LDL cholesterol levels by 6 percent, despite having eaten more fat each day than the control subjects.

Mavis Abbey, M.D., at the division of human nutrition, Commonwealth Scientific and Industrial Research Organization, Australia, studied the effects of various nuts on sixteen men with normal cholesterol levels. Abbey found that not all fats are alike. Using almonds, walnuts, peanuts (not a true nut), and coconut, during a nine-week study, the men ate a typical high-fat (36 percent) Australian diet. In the first three-week period, used as a reference period, half of the 36 percent of dietary fat came from raw peanuts, coconut cubes, and a coconut confectionery bar. During the second three-week period, the men ate almonds instead of peanuts, and coconut cubes and bars. In the final three-week period, walnuts were substituted for almonds and comprised up to 18 percent of the dietary fat. In comparison to the reference period of peanuts and coconut, after eating almonds for three weeks, total cholesterol levels declined 7 percent; and with walnuts, declined 5 percent. The decline resulted from lower LDL cholesterol levels. LDL levels were 10 percent lower in the group eating almonds and 9 percent lower in the group eating walnuts. The HDL levels did not decline.

Abbey commented that "dietary studies have usually used dietary oils as the source of polyunsaturated and monounsaturated fatty acids. Very little work has been done in which specific foods have been examined for their effect on plasma lipids and coronary heart disease outcomes." (*American Journal of Clinical Nutrition*, 1994; 59: 995–999)

Nuts may reduce the risk of stroke. Walnuts are especially rich in alpha-linolenic acid, as mentioned earlier. Researchers at the University of California in San Francisco, led by Joel Simon, M.D., M.P.H., found that the higher the level of this fatty acid in the blood, the lower was the risk of stroke.

Simon reported that "alpha-linolenic acid is converted in the body into omega-3 fatty acid, the same kind that is in fish oil. And there's good evidence that fish oil discourages the formation of blood clots. So eating walnuts may be another way to get the [same] benefits of fish oil." (*Health*, July/Aug 1996: 36)

The overwhelming evidence demonstrates that, for years, the conventional wisdom that all high-fat foods promote plaque and lead to arterial and cardiovascular diseases was wrong. Numerous investigations, as demonstrated, show that foods rich in monounsaturated fatty acids, such as nuts, actually lower the risks, and in some cases, are even more effective in doing so than the standard low-fat diet recommended by the American Heart Association (AHA) and other groups, including governmental agencies.

Nuts and Cancer

Relatively less research effort has been given to the potential role of nuts in reducing cancer risk. However, the few studies that exist show promise.

One study, led by John Milner, Ph.D., and Penny Kris-Etherton, Ph.D., professors of nutrition at Pennsylvania State University at State College, Pennsylvania, showed that phytochemicals in almonds inhibited the growth of tumor cells maintained in laboratory culture. Two flavonoid compounds, quercetin and kaempherol were identified as especially strong suppressors of lung and prostate tumor cell growth.

Elsewhere, two published studies examined nut consumption and prostate cancer. The first study showed a decreased risk of prostate cancer with an increased intake of nuts, beans, and lentils. The other study, published in the *Journal of the National Cancer Institute* in 2000, included data for men forty-five to seventy-four years of age from fifty-nine different countries. Their death rate from prostate cancer decreased as their consumption of nuts and seeds increased. Often, zinc-rich pumpkin seeds are included in diets to promote prostate health.

In a test to learn whether nuts play any role in preventing colon cancer, Dr. Paul A. Davis, whose work was discussed previously, chose rats that were predisposed to develop colon cancer. Davis fed a control group a diet with cellulose (an indigestible insoluble fiber with no nutrients), and fed another group a diet containing 20 percent almonds. All of the rats developed aberrant crypt foci (ACFs), considered to be early markers for colon tumor development. However, the rats fed almonds in their diet developed far fewer ACFs than did the control group on the diet with cellulose. Davis told *Food Product Design* in July 1999 that, "almonds appear to inhibit the formation of ACFs, precancerous lesions, which are red flags for colon cancer."

Nuts and Obesity

It may sound like an oxymoron to suggest that a high-fat food such as nuts might be appropriate in a weight-reduction diet. However, nuts do not lead to weight gain. In fact, they may help people adhere better and longer to weight-loss programs, according to the findings of a study conducted by Kathy McManus, R.D., director of nutrition at Brigham and Women's Hospital in Boston. McManus placed participants on two different weight-loss programs, which they were to follow for eighteen months. One plan was a low-fat diet, and the other, a moderate-fat diet. In the moderate-fat diet, participants could snack on any nuts of their choosing. The participants lost about ten pounds on both plans during the first period. However, after one year, participants on the low-fat diet found compliance somewhat difficult, and they began to gain some weight. The participants on the moderate-fat diet with the addition of nuts maintained their weight loss. Also, more subjects on this diet adhered to the program for the full eighteen months of the study.

For years, the conventional wisdom had been that nuts, as high-fat foods, contribute to obesity—quite the contrary, judging from the results of several studies. Frank Sacks, M.D., associate professor of medicine at the Harvard School of Public Health in Boston, conducted studies with 101 overweight individuals who repeatedly failed to reduce weight following traditional weight-reduction diets. The participants in Sacks's study, mostly women, averaged about 200 pounds each at the beginning of the study.

Using guidelines offered by the researchers, the participants prepared their own meals. Half of the participants were assigned to a diet in which 35 percent of calories were from monounsaturated fats, with added nuts, peanuts, and olives, as well as selected oils. The other half ate a diet containing only 20 percent fats—a typical low-fat diet.

Within three months, both groups lost from five to thirty pounds, and then stabilized. After six months, 62 percent of the dieters eating the higher-fat diet continued to adhere to the plan. Only 45 percent of those on the low-fat diet remained in compliance. The high-fat diet was more palatable, offered more satiety, and thereby resulted in more weight loss. The low-fat diet, less appetizing and providing less satiety, was difficult to maintain.

Sacks's work was strengthened by studies conducted elsewhere. Richard

Mattes, Ph.D., R.D., at Purdue University in West Lafayette, Indiana, demonstrated that the addition of nuts to the diet did not interfere with weight-loss programs. People following such diets compensated calorically for the nuts. "It appears that these people are calorically compensating for the nuts beautifully... their body weights are staying remarkable stable." (*Science News,* 21 Nov 1998: 330)

Several of the studies discussed in the section on the cardiovascular benefits of nuts also showed that nut consumption did not lead to weight gain. Most consumers of nuts in the Loma Linda study were thinner than those who did not eat nuts. In Dr. Spiller's studies, volunteers ate 3.5 ounces of almonds daily—590 calories, the equivalent of two big scoops of ice cream. Yet, at the end of nine weeks, the volunteers did not gain any weight. Spiller concluded that the participants did not gain weight because nuts, dense in nutrients, satisfy hunger pangs and thereby reduce the number of total calories consumed.

DISTINGUISHING THE NUTS

All nuts are nutritious, but each type has specific characteristics. You may enjoy some more than others. However, it is wise to add as much variety as you can. This practice allows you to obtain the special benefits from different types of nuts. It also minimizes the possible buildup of allergic reactions that can result from eating the same food, repeatedly, over time.

Almonds

The almond has a venerable history. It is mentioned seventy-three times in the Old Testament. The almond was cultivated in Asia Minor and the Mediterranean basin, long before the Christian era. Middle Easterners were probably the first people to use almonds as a regular staple in their diets. By the Middle Ages, they spread the cultivation of almond trees as they expanded the boundaries of Islam to Spain. The colonial expansion of Spain took almond trees to the New World, with the planting of almond trees in California's Spanish missions. Now, several centuries later, almonds are California's largest tree crop, and the state is the world's leading almond producer.

What is special about almonds? Of all nuts, the fatty acid composition of the almond is most like that of olive oil, with a high proportion of MUFAs and smaller proportions of PUFAs and SFAs.

The almond is an outstanding source of alpha-tocopherol (one form of vitamin E), a valuable antioxidant. About 1 ounce ($\frac{1}{4}$ cup) of almonds provide 10 international units (IU) of vitamin E. A study funded by the National Institutes of Health and published in the *New England Journal of Medicine* showed that alpha-tocopherol is the form of vitamin E that is best absorbed and utilized. This vitamin promotes cardiovascular health and, in conjunction with the polyphenols also present in almonds, may reduce the risk of certain cancers and boost the immune system. Also, there is some evidence that this vitamin is an anti-inflammatory agent. Consumers value this vitamin for its antiaging properties. By making skin more supple, it gives a more youthful appearance.

The phytochemicals in almonds include several other antioxidants: the flavonoid quercetin, as well as caffeic and ferulic acids. At least twelve flavonoids have been identified in almond protein, and five more have been detected but, to date, not identified. Almonds also contain phytosterols such as beta-sitosterol, which is reported to lower blood cholesterol without lowering HDL levels. Also present is benzaldehyde, whose anti-inflammatory properties (in addition to those of vitamin E) might benefit arthritics and others. Benzaldehyde is an aromatic oil present in bitter almonds.

A study at Tufts University suggested that the nutrients found in the pellicle (skin) of the almond, together with the nut, may offer a significantly higher amount of health benefits than when these nutrients are isolated from each other. Therefore, it is better to eat almonds that have not been blanched.

Brazil Nuts

Most Brazil nuts come from trees that grow wild in the dense tropical jungles of the Brazilian states and territories of the Amazon River basin, as well as from some commercial plantations. The tree thrives in hot, humid, and rainy weather. Attempts to cultivate the Brazil tree in other parts of the world have not been successful.

Studies show that the entire nut tree, its bark, trunk, and roots, as well as its nuts, all contain relatively high concentrations of radium compared to other foods. One of the chemical elements essential to the Brazil nut tree is barium, a trace mineral. Because the soil in the Amazon basin is deficient in barium, the tree takes up radium as a substitute. However, even if an adult eats an ounce (about $1/4$ cup) of Brazil nuts daily, exposure to radium is only about 7 percent of the average total dose of radium received daily from natural background sources.

The Brazil nut is a good source of selenium, which works in tandem with vitamin E. The Brazil nut has about equal parts of MUFAs and PUFAs, and far less of SFAs.

Cashews

The cashew is native to Brazil and cultivated in many tropical countries. Portuguese explorers carried cashews from Brazil to India in the sixteenth century. Cashews proved to be highly adapted to South India and East Africa. Currently, cashews are imported from India, Africa, Brazil, and Indonesia. Very few are grown in the United States.

The cashew tree belongs to the same family of plants as those species that cause poison ivy, poison oak, and poison sumac. The tree itself bears a pear-shaped fruit called the cashew apple. Unlike other nuts, the cashew nut grows on the distal, or flower, end of the fruit, rather than being encased in the fruit's pulp. The nut is composed of an inner kernel and a double-layered outer shell. Between the layers of shell is an oil containing at least twelve chemically distinct antigens (substances that can induce antibody formation and have irritating and allergenic properties). Workers who shell cashews manually commonly develop *pruritus dermatitis* (severe itching of the skin). Outbreaks have occurred, too, among dockworkers unloading whole, unprocessed cashews. *Vesicular dermatitis* (skin irritation that produces cysts) was reported among children who played with souvenir toy burros made from cashews shells wired together with beads. Modern processing equipment has reduced the frequency of this problem among workers handling cashews in the shell. Cashew nuts are processed to remove the shells and oils before the nuts are roasted and sold. Some cashew nuts, which are very lightly roasted and appear white, sometimes are mislabeled as raw nuts.

Cashews are a good source of copper, iron, and folacin, in addition to other nutrients, fiber, and phytochemicals.

Chestnuts

Nearly all trees of the American chestnut have been destroyed by fungus blight. Chinese chestnut trees, which are blight resistant, are sold in place of the American chestnut for yard and orchard culture. Some Japanese chestnuts are imported from Japan and some are grown in the United States, but they are not as well adapted to the North American climate as are the Chinese chestnuts. European or Italian chestnuts are available in American markets around the holiday season. Also, in some cities, chestnuts are roasted and sold in streets.

The chestnut is the only low-fat nut and has fewer calories than other nuts. It is rich in fiber. One cup of shelled chestnuts contains about 310 calories. Over 85 percent are from carbohydrates and the remaining 15 percent is divided equally between protein and fat. Chestnuts provide a generous amount of potassium and smaller amounts of B vitamins and iron.

In selecting chestnuts, squeeze hard. If you feel some space, the chestnuts may not be fresh. When pressed, the chestnuts should be flush against the shells. Discard any that are moldy or shriveled. Do not eat them raw. Like other highly starchy foods (for example, potatoes), chestnuts need to be cooked before they are consumed.

Coconut

It is thought that the coconut played a significant role in the diet of our pre-agricultural ancestors. The coconut "meat" (pulp) was eaten in ancient Greece, and its "milk" (liquid) was also consumed. Both pulp and liquid were consumed in ancient times by people of the Indus Valley in Asia. By the mid-thirteenth century, Chinese writers described coconut meat as being of "a jade-like white and of an agreeable taste, resembling that of cow's milk." (*Food in History*, Stein & Day, 1973)

When Portuguese explorers sailed to the Indian Ocean in 1499, they brought fresh coconuts back to Europe. Because coconuts can be transported readily by sea or by land, coconuts were spread globally from the European colonial lands, especially to tropical East Africa and Latin America.

Not only was the coconut consumed, but also its oil provided a hair unguent, a body emollient, an iron rust inhibitor, a lamp fuel, a textile-mill lubricant, and an ingredient for soap making. The oil supplanted animal fats for soap making. By doing so, it led to the establishment of fish-and-chip shops in England. Coconut oil, being white, odorless, and stable, did not splatter in frying and could be strained and reused.

You may enjoy eating coconut but are discouraged from buying whole coconuts because of the difficulty in cracking open the hard shell to extract the meat. However, the effort is worthwhile. You can pierce the two "eyes" (the dark circles) with a strong instrument such as a clean screwdriver, tapped at its end with a hammer. After you pierce the holes, drain the milk into a container and drink it. Place the coconut on a wooden board or, if possible, on a grassy area outdoors, and split the shell with a hammer. Extract the pieces with a strong knife.

Compared to other nuts, coconut is relatively low in protein. However, it has other virtues. It provides calcium, iron, magnesium, phosphorus, and potassium, as well as iodine and many other micronutrients. The coconut consists of about 60 percent fat, which is predominantly saturated. The main fatty acid in coconut is lauric acid (45 percent). The other main fatty acids are myristic, 18 percent; palmitic, 9 percent; oleic, 8 percent; caprylic and capric, 7 percent each; and stearic, 5 percent. A medium-sized coconut, weighing about 14 ounces, contains 13 milligrams (mg) of vitamin C. It contains some tocopherol (vitamin E), and a mature coconut is a good source of fiber (35 grams).

A major contribution of the coconut is its lauric acid. This beneficial medium-chain fatty acid has potent antiviral, antifungal, and antimicrobial properties. In laboratory tests, lauric acid was shown to be capable of inactivating many important and some potentially life-threatening viruses, including HIV, measles, herpes simplex, vesicular stomatitis, visna, and cytomegalovirus.

Hazelnuts

Although we tend to use the names hazelnut and filbert interchangeably, there are distinctions. Hazelnuts are from a tree native to North America, and many grow wild. The nuts from cultivated European species are known as filberts: the giant filbert and the European filbert. Hazelnuts are grown in Oregon and the State of Washington. Also, they are imported from Turkey, Italy, and Spain.

The ancient Chinese regarded the hazelnut as one of the five "sacred nourishments" bestowed on human beings. The Chinese have cultivated hazelnuts continuously for more than 4,500 years.

It is thought that the nut acquired the name filbert because August 20, the day when the nut is supposed to start ripening, coincided with St. Philibert's Day.

Hazelnuts are a good source of vitamin E; vitamins B_2, B_3, B_6, and folacin in the vitamin B complex; as well as calcium, iron, copper, magnesium, phosphorus, potassium, biotin, and dietary fiber. The fatty acids in the hazelnut have a composition quite similar to that of olive oil.

Macadamias

The macadamia tree was first described scientifically in the mid-nineteenth century by the Australian botanist Baron Ferdinand von Mueller, who named it to honor a friend, Dr. John Macadam.

The macadamia tree is native to Australia, but we generally associate its production with Hawaii. Both Australia and Hawaii are major exporters of macadamia nuts. Other countries where the nut grows include South Africa, China, Malaysia, Guatemala, Costa Rica, and Brazil.

Unlike other nuts that have one harvest time of ripening, macadamias ripen at intervals and need to have the harvest repeated five or six times. Manual harvesting and the difficulty of removing an extraordinarily hard shell make these nuts expensive. Also, it takes about seven years for newly planted trees to bear a supply of nuts, and five to eight years more for a larger supply. This factor, too, makes the nut expensive. However, the trees live for about fifty to a hundred years and continue to be productive.

Of all nuts, macadamias are the richest tasting, because they have the highest level of fat (59 percent). Most of the fat is monounsaturated. Macadamia nuts contribute a fair amount of magnesium, iron, and thiamine (vitamin B_1) to the diet.

Pecans

The pecan is native to temperate North America. Records of the Spanish conquistadors DeSoto and de Oviedo reveal that Native Americans had been using nuts of the "pacan" tree long before Europeans arrived on these shores.

Pecan trees grow wild from Illinois to the Gulf Coast. The largest nut forests are found along the riverbanks of the lower Mississippi Valley. Nuts from these trees are quite small and have hard shells.

Georgia is the leading state producing cultivated pecans. Other states include Texas, the Carolinas, Florida, Arizona, and New Mexico. Mexico, Brazil, Australia, South Africa, and Israel also produce pecans.

A study in 2002, reported in the *Journal of Food Science,* showed that no matter the variety or the region in which pecans are grown, their content of vitamin E remains abundant and constant. Pecans contain both the alpha- and gamma-tocopherol forms of vitamin E. According to Ron Eitenmiller, Ph.D., a food scientist at the College of Agricultural and Environmental Sciences at the University of Georgia at Athens, "Vitamin E is the principal antioxidant we use. It protects our bodies when chemical reactions produce oxidation in the body, which can be dangerous. Antioxidants, in essence, serve as a tool that inhibits oxidative stress that can be detrimental to many cellular functions."

Vitamin E is not produced by our bodies. Our supply must come from foods. All nuts are good sources of vitamin E.

Pecans have at least nineteen vitamins and minerals that, to date, have been identified. They are good sources of folic acid, calcium, magnesium, copper, potassium, manganese, and zinc. Pecans also are a good source of plant sterols.

Pine Nuts

The pignolia (also known as European pine nut, pignoli, pignon, piñon nut, and Indian nut) has a venerable history. Remains of it have been found in ancient Roman and Greek ruins. The European pine nut is richer in protein than any other nut or seed. The pinyon (or piñon) is native to the American Southwest and has been part of the Native American diet for thousands of years. Pine nuts come from pinecones of trees of the genus *Pinus*. Edible wild species require painstaking hand labors and are extremely expensive.

The pignolia contains less fat than the pinyon. One ounce (approximately $1/4$ cup) of pignolia contains 14 grams of fat; pinyon, 17 grams. Pine nuts contribute a fair amount of magnesium, iron, and vitamin B_1 to the diet.

Pine nuts most commonly sold in the United States are imported from Turkey and China. The smooth cones are opened by sun drying, and each seed is removed manually. Once the pine trees bearing pignolias are cultivated, it takes a quarter of a century before the first crop may be gathered. Full production is not reached until about seventy-five years. Crops appear only once every five to seven years. Piñon gathering and shelling is difficult and labor intensive. All of these factors account for the irregular appearance of these nuts in the marketplace, and their high cost.

Pistachios

The birthplace of the pistachio can be traced back to the holy lands of the Middle East, where originally pistachio trees grew wild in high-desert regions. Modern times has seen the nut cultivated in Iran, Turkey, Syria, Greece, and Italy, before becoming a major crop in California. When pistachios were still being imported, they were obtained mostly from the Middle East. American importers dyed the shells red, both to attract the attention of potential buyers and also to cover blemishes caused by antiquated harvesting methods. Currently, red-shelled pistachios are out of favor. Only about 1 percent of pistachio shells continue to be dyed, by use of a cornstarch-base red color, allura red (FD&C Red No. 40). Pistachios are a good source of iron, copper, phosphorus, and vitamin B_1. A $1/4$ cup (1 ounce) serving of pistachios contains more than 10 percent of the daily value of fiber. Surprisingly, there is more fiber in a serving of pistachios than in a half-cup serving of broccoli.

Walnuts

Commonly, English or Persian walnuts are simply called walnuts. Because they originated in Persia they were first called Persian walnuts. After they were introduced to England, and then brought to America, they were called English walnuts. Today, California is the center of commercial walnut production in the United States.

The ancient Romans considered certain nuts to be foods of the gods. The walnut was one. During the Renaissance, walnuts were used to treat head ailments because the physical appearance of walnuts resembles the brain.

According to the American Dietetic Association (ADA), an ounce (approximately $\frac{1}{4}$ cup) of walnuts supplies about 2 grams of plant-based omega-3 fatty acids. This beneficial substance may account for anti-inflammatory properties in walnuts, as identified by researchers at the University of California at Davis.

Walnuts contain protective natural antioxidants. These include both alpha- and gamma-tocopherols, as well as ellagic acid.

Inside the walnut shell, the kernels are surrounded by the pellicle, a special protective coating. The pellicle is rich in several compounds that help protect the nut against oxidation. When the kernels are broken into pieces, their unsaturated fatty acids are exposed to more oxygen, which accelerates rancidity. Therefore, it is best to select intact kernels.

BUYING AND STORING NUTS

Nuts with their shells intact keep longer than shelled nuts, because the shells prevent damage from air and prevent oxidation and rancidity. Pistachios are easy to shell because the roasting process splits them open partially. Some nuts, such as almonds, walnuts, pecans, and hazelnuts, are relatively easy to shell by using a manual nutcracker and nut pick. Other nuts, such as Brazil nuts, are difficult to shell unless you use a special device. Cashews and macadamias are sold already shelled. As mentioned earlier, the cashew shell contains irritating caustics, and the macadamias have extremely hard shells.

If you wish to purchase nuts still encased in their shells, look for ones that are clean, uncracked, and heavy. The availability of good nut-cracking devices intended for home use has dwindled considerably. Appliances, formerly long available, are no longer being manufactured. In this age of convenience, shelling nuts has gone out of favor. However, at least one manufacturer continues to produce a sturdy nutcracker that can be used with all nuts, even those that are challenging. That product is Krakanut, manufactured by Felko Products, Inc. (3380 Texas South, Minneapolis, Minnesota 55426; (952) 935-3758; www.krakanut.com).

If you buy nuts already shelled, the best supplies are available from health/natural food stores. Usually, they are prepackaged and refrigerated.

Some are vacuum-packed. If there is a rapid turnover of stock in bulk bins, the nuts may be fresh. Judge by smelling and sampling. Some types of nuts turn rancid quickly; examples are pecans and pignolias. Other types stay fresh longer; examples are almonds and filberts. Avoid purchasing broken nuts.

Most nuts are roasted before they are sold. Because nuts are already rich in oil, "dry roasting" is a gimmick. Oil roasting of nuts adds only a negligible amount of additional oil. However, some of the oils used for roasting (such as cottonseed oil) are undesirable.

Salted nuts contain about 200 milligrams of sodium per serving. Unsalted and lightly salted nuts contain less than 60 milligrams of sodium per serving. Often, you have a choice of salted or unsalted nuts.

At home, transfer the nuts purchased from bulk bins into tightly closed containers, preferably glass, up to the top of the containers to keep out as much air as possible. If space permits, shelled or unshelled nuts are best stored in the freezer. You can remove small quantities of nuts from the freezer for immediate use, because nuts thaw out in several minutes. As the supply of nuts in the freezer is used, and there is headspace in the containers, transfer the nuts to smaller and smaller containers, to exclude as much air as possible. This also frees more freezer space for other items.

If freezer space is too limited for nut storage, store them in the coldest section of the refrigerator. Use the same method for air exclusion as in the freezer.

Nuts Are Not for Everyone

Although most people tolerate nuts well, some people do not. Tree nuts are among the most common allergens. Some people need to avoid all nuts; others, only specific ones. It is helpful to know which botanical family is involved. Nuts are often linked not only with other nuts but also with other types of food in the same botanical family. For example, the cashew family includes not only the cashew nut, but also the pistachio and the mango. If an individual has an allergic reaction to one of these foods, he or she likely reacts unfavorably to the other foods in the same family. Both the beechnut and the chestnut are in the beech family; hazelnut (filbert) and oil of birch are in the birch family; pinyon (piñon) pine nut and juniper are in the pine family; almond, apricot, cherry, peach, plum (and prune), and nectarine are in the plum family; and pecan, butternut, hickory, and walnut (both black and English) are in the walnut family. Coconut, along with date, palm cabbage, and sago, are in the palm family. Neither the Brazil nut in the lecythis family, nor the macadamia nut in the macadamia family, shares any food-family associations.

Individuals who know that they are allergic to specific nuts can recognize them as whole nuts and avoid them. However, eating foods prepared by others, either processed foods or food eaten when away from home, may be hazardous. Frequently, nuts are hidden and unsuspected ingredients. For a nut-allergic person, the consequences can be serious, or even fatal. Label reading is important but fails to offer adequate protection. The safest solution is to prepare all foods consumed and to shun all prepared by others. This measure sounds draconian, but it saves lives.

The development of bioengineered foods adds a new dimension to food allergy. Components of foods introduced into other foods may create hazards for some people. The case of Brazil nuts may be a harbinger. A genetic engineering company in Iowa developed a transgenic soybean containing methionine-rich 2S albumin from the Brazil nut. Soybeans lack methionine, an essential amino acid, and the attempt to introduce methionine from the Brazil nut might correct the deficiency. Although the Food and Drug Administration (FDA) had devised a policy on transgenic (cross-breed) plant foods as early as 1992, the rules require notification and testing only for foods with genes transferred from the major common allergies. The list does not include Brazil nuts or many other food allergens.

The genetic engineering company consulted the FDA about the need for premarketing safety tests of its transgenic soybean. The research scientists who conducted the tests demonstrated that people who react to Brazil-nut extracts on standard skin-prick tests also react to extracts of the transgenic soybean. This finding demonstrated that an allergen from a food known to be allergenic can be transferred to a new food by genetic engineering. Once the findings on the allergenicity of the new product were established, the company had the choice of labeling the new soybeans as allergenic or of withdrawing the product from the marketplace. The company chose to withdraw the product. (*New England Journal of Medicine,* 14 Mar 1996; 334 [11]: 688–692; also editorial: 726–728)

SEEDS: THE GERM OF LIFE

Seeds, like nuts, are dense in nutrients, fiber, and beneficial phytochemicals. Some edible seeds are used as flavorings (dill, poppy, and cumin); some, as digestives (caraway, anise, and fennel); and some, as whole foods in the diet (sunflower, pumpkin, sesame, and flaxseeds).

Flaxseeds

The flax plant is one of the oldest known cultivated plants, probably originating in Asia. According to archaeological evidence, flax was cultivated in Babylon around 5000 B.C. Flaxseeds and seed pods, wall paintings depicting the seed's cultivation, and cloth made from flax fibers (linen) were found in the oldest known burial chambers of the Egyptians, from about 3000 B.C. Both flaxseeds and flax fibers were found in archaeological digs in Switzerland from the late Stone Age, about 4000 to 3000 B.C.

The ancient Greeks and Romans were aware of the healing properties of flax as early as about 650 B.C. In the fifth century B.C., Hippocrates, the ancient Greek physician revered as the "Father of Medicine," mentioned the use of flax to relieve inflammation of mucous membranes, abdominal pain, and diarrhea. Theophrastus used the mucilage, formed by soaking flaxseeds, to relieve coughs. The historian Tacitus, in the first century of the Christian era, praised flax in his writings. By the eighth century, Emperor Charlemagne considered flaxseed so vital to the health of his subjects that he formulated regulations requiring its consumption.

In Europe, through the centuries, flax was cultivated for its seeds as well as for its oil and fiber. In modern times, Mahatma Gandhi observed, "Wherever flaxseed becomes a regular food item among the people, there will be better health."

Unfortunately, after World War II, flaxseed was nearly forgotten. Large oil mills pressed oil seeds that were more stable than flax, but inferior in their health benefits. The textile industry abandoned linen manufacture from flax and embraced nylon, polyester, and other synthetics. The paint industry rejected linseed oil (made from flax oil) and favored man-made drying oils.

Fortunately, interest in flaxseed has revived, due to the rediscovery of its benefits and the discovery of phytochemicals in foods. Currently, flax is grown globally in temperate climates. The main suppliers are Argentina, India, and the United States. Also, it is grown in Canada, many European countries, Russia, China, Egypt, and Morocco.

Although the nutritional value of flaxseed varies slightly from year to year, and depending on the growing area, a sample of 100 grams of seeds yields, on average, about 45 grams of oil, 22 grams of protein, and 12 grams of fiber. The cooler the climate where the plant is grown, the higher will be the oil content in the seed.

The flaxseed is one whole food that you should *not* eat whole. Whole flaxseeds merely go through the intestinal tract intact, and you derive no benefit from them. In order to obtain the nutrients from flaxseeds, you need to crush them. You can use a mortar and pestle, an electric seed grinder, an electric blender, or a food processor. However, you must do the grinding *immediately* before you intend to use the ground flaxseed meal. The oil in the seed is highly perishable and begins to deteriorate quickly after the seed is crushed.

The oil in flaxseed is of the very highest quality—possibly the best of any food seed. As noted in Chapter 1, in the discussion of salad dressings, the flaxseed oil is very rich in both alpha-linolenic (omega-3) and linoleic (omega-6) acids—two essential fatty acids. On average, flaxseed oil contains 54 percent omega-3 fatty acids, 15 percent omega-6 fatty acids, and 21 percent of the nonessential but highly beneficial omega-9 fatty acids. The remainder of the oil contents consists of nonessential unsaturates, oleic acid, and some SFAs.

Among all seed oils, the oil from flaxseed has a unique feature. It contains a substance that resembles prostaglandins, which regulate blood pressure and arterial functions. Also, prostaglandins are important in calcium and energy metabolism.

The oil in flaxseed is rich in phosphatides, including lecithin. The phosphatides help digest fats and oils. Flaxseed oil also contains carotene and vitamin E, as well as a wide range of proteins, minerals, and other vitamins.

Flaxseed oil is highly perishable. It should be stored in a dark container. Once the container is unsealed, close it tightly and refrigerate. Purchase it in quantities that you can use within a reasonable period of time.

After stressing the importance of grinding flaxseeds before using them, mention must be made of one exception! When whole flaxseeds are moistened, they swell and form a mucilage around them. This mucilage is helpful in relieving constipation. The whole flaxseeds, in absorbing water, swell to about three times their dry volume and become encased in the mucilage. If accompanied by lots of additional fluid, the mucilage provides a natural laxative with no side effects (unless one is allergic to flaxseed). The mucilage also buffers the effects of excessive stomach acidity. The mucilage is capable of lowering blood cholesterol by preventing the bile acids from being reabsorbed, decreases absorption of cholesterol from foods, and increases the amount of cholesterol excreted. The mucilage also helps to stabilize and modulate blood glucose.

Store flaxseeds properly. The intact seeds are stable, provided you keep them in a tightly closed container and exclude as much air as possible. The seeds will keep for a long time in a cool, dry place. Even better, store them either in the freezer or refrigerator.

After you grind the flaxseeds, you can use them in many ways. Add them to cereal, soup, stew, or casserole dishes.

Pumpkin Seeds

Hulled, green pumpkin seeds (sometimes called *pepitas*) are an ancient variety of pumpkin. They are available in vacuum-packed bags in some food stores, and loose in bins in many health/natural food stores. Many are imported from China.

Pumpkin seeds are good sources of healthful fats. They are high in potassium, magnesium, phosphorus, calcium, sodium, zinc, iron, and copper. Few studies have been conducted, but the oil contained in the seeds, as well as their zinc content, appear to be helpful in reducing symptoms of benign prostatic hyperplasia (prostate gland enlargement), especially when they are used in combination with saw palmetto.

Squash seeds, the crunchy white pumpkin seeds with their hulls intact, are eaten mainly for the hulls. There is little seed content within the hulls. The hulls provide a good source of fiber.

The Navajo Indians, especially, prepared whole squash seeds by roasting and salting them. The Pima Indians regarded squash seeds as a delicacy. They parched them by placing the seeds in ollas (ceramic storage containers) with live coals, and stirred them until the seeds were roasted thoroughly.

Sesame Seeds

Sesame seeds have a venerable history. The ancient Assyrians recorded stories of their gods drinking sesame wine the night before they created the earth. Numerous archaeological digs have uncovered evidence that oil from the sesame seed was used thousands of years before the Christian era. The Babylonians made cakes, as well as wine and brandy, from sesame seeds. They used the oil for cooking, for toiletries such as perfume, and for medicinal purposes, including its use for reptile bites.

Many years later, African slaves brought sesame seeds and sesame oil to America. In the Bantu dialect, sesame seed was known as "benne." This term is still used for sesame seeds in cities such as Charleston, South Carolina, and New Orleans, Louisiana.

Sesame seeds come from an annual plant that is at least six feet tall. It grows well in fertile, well-drained soil, in warm climates. The seeds are oval-shaped and covered by fibrous hulls that range in color from light tan, to yellowish white, to red, brown, and black. Seeds imported to the United States usually are light tan. When the hull is removed, the seed is white and glossy.

Sesame seed plants are native to East Africa, India, Afghanistan, and Indonesia. The plants are grown in those areas, as well as in Mexico, Central America, and northern South America. Some plants are grown in the United States, mainly in Texas and Oklahoma. Our major import suppliers are Mexico, Guatemala, Nicaragua, El Salvador, Venezuela, and India.

The sesame seed contains between 50 and 60 percent oil, which is low in SFAs. The seed has antioxidants that help maintain the oil's stability. The oil from the sesame seed is highly valued, and it ranks sixth in world production of edible oil seeds.

Sesame seeds are comparatively high in calcium and vitamin B. They contain about 25 to 30 percent protein, including sulfur-based amino acids such as methionine and cystine—two amino acids lacking in many other plant sources.

The oil in unhulled sesame seeds is quite stable, and the seeds have a relatively long shelf life. Unhulled seeds will keep well stored at room temperature for up to two years. After hulling, sesame seeds have a far shorter shelf life. Such seeds need to be refrigerated. Also, the hulling should be done mechanically, not with harsh caustics.

Because of their diminutive size, sesame seeds are generally not eaten out of the hand, because they cannot be managed as readily as sunflower or pumpkin seeds, or nuts. However, they can be sprinkled over vegetable or fruit salads, used to top casseroles, baked fish, or poached eggs, or added to baked goods.

Unfortunately, sesame seeds cannot be tolerated by everyone. In sensitized individuals, sesame seeds can provoke serious allergic reactions, including urticaria (skin wheals or welts, accompanied by severe itching), Quincke's edema (recurrent attacks of an abnormal accumulation of fluid in intercellular spaces of the body, suddenly appearing in areas of the skin or mucous membranes, and occasionally in the viscera or major internal organs), asthma, and even anaphylactic shock. Some respiratory distress and urticaria result from exposure to, and inhalation of, sesame-seed dust by workers. "Baker's asthma," an occupational hazard, can be triggered by repeated exposure to sesame seeds. (See *Allergy,* January 1996, vol. 51, no. 1, pp. 69–70.)

Other cases of sesame-seed allergy have resulted from the seeds being added to foods. As the seeds have become more popular, they are being used in ever more food products. When they appear in the form of ground meal, they are no longer recognizable as the whole seeds and are, therefore, hidden allergens.

A 1996 study of the prevalence of allergic reactions to foods by young children, conducted at the Royal Children's Hospital in Melbourne, Australia, indicated that sensitization to sesame seeds was becoming more common. This was reflected by an increase in infantile eczema and anaphylaxis after the allergic children ate foods with sesame seeds, such as tahini (ground, hulled sesame seeds), dips, and vegetable burgers, which had become a larger part of the Australian diet. (*British Medical Journal*, 7 Dec 1996: 313 [7070]: 1477–1478)

The allergens in sesame seeds can be inactivated or destroyed by thorough heating of the seeds.

Sunflower Seeds

The wild sunflower plant is native to the Americas. In the American Southwest, since prehistoric times, Native Americans cultivated single-headed sunflower plants. They gathered the seeds, parched them, and sometimes ate them whole. Apparently, the shells were thin enough to eat. Also, the people ground the seeds into meal.

The Spanish conquistadors found that the sunflower plant was important in Central and South America, both as food and as part of religious rituals. Reproductions of sunflowers, sculpted in gold, were found in Inca temples. Elsewhere, Native Americans showed colonial settlers from Europe how to use sunflower seeds as food.

Native Americans continued to grow their own hardy indigenous varieties of sunflower seeds. From various parts of the plant, they made black, purple, and yellow dyes for clothing and baskets, and they shredded the stalks to make fiber twine for nets.

The sunflower plant has been used, too, for medicines. Old herbal books record its use as a diuretic and expectorant, and for treatment of bronchial and pulmonary problems, coughs, colds, and pertussis. The root of the plant was used to treat snakebites, and the astringent leaves were used as an herbal tobacco.

Currently, two different types of sunflower plants are raised for food use. One is for oil extraction; the other, for seed use. Both types have flowers with bright yellow petals. However, the sunflowers intended for oil extraction have small black seeds; those for edible seeds have larger kernels, and the hulls are gray with white stripes. The smaller ones intended as edible seeds are used in bird feed.

The raw kernel is exceptionally stable, keeping its freshness for about a year. Roasted kernels show some rancidity after about three months of storage at room temperature and when they are exposed to air. Therefore, purchase sunflowers only in quantities that you can use within a limited time. If they are vacuum-packed, the air has been excluded. However, if they are sold loose, they should be refrigerated in the store, not in bins where they are exposed to air and are at room temperature. Unless there is a very rapid turnover, sunflower seeds stored under such conditions may be rancid. The odor of mild rancidity is not detected readily, but it is toxic. At home, keep the vacuum-packaged seeds in a cool, dry place. Transfer those purchased in bulk bins and packaged in bags to containers. Fill to the top and either freeze or refrigerate them, following the same procedures discussed earlier with nuts.

Sunflower seeds are high in vitamin E, linoleic acid (omega-6), zinc, iron, and dietary fiber. They are a good source of vitamin D, not found in many plant sources. They consist of approximately 50 percent fat: the majority is PUFAs, with lesser amounts of MUFAs and SFAs. On average, their protein content is comparable to that of peanuts. They are a good source of several vitamin B fractions: thiamine (vitamin B_1), riboflavin (vitamin B_2), niacin (vitamin B_3), and folate. They are also a good source of vitamin A. They contain calcium, potassium, magnesium, phosphorus, and fluorine. Sunflower seeds contain several polyphenol compounds: chlorogenic, caffeic, and quinic acids.

Due largely to recent medical and nutritional research projects, nuts and seeds have achieved a new and deserved elevated status. No longer are they regarded as high-fat, high-caloric foods that need to be consumed sparingly, possibly as food garnishes. Nuts and seeds are nutrient dense and they have quality oils and phytonutrients that contribute to good health. As whole foods, they can be used and enjoyed frequently and are beneficial for most people.

CHAPTER 5

Quality Counts
with Protein Foods

protein: from the Greek protos, *meaning first*
protein: from late Greek proteios, *meaning of the first quality*

As we will discuss in this chapter, not all protein foods are created equal. Some are better balanced than others due to their amino acid composition. Eggs, for example, have greater protein value than beans. Because protein is so important to our health, it is crucial that we seek out quality protein foods.

Protein was the first substance identified as an essential part of living tissue. The name, derived from Greek, means "of primary importance." Protein is the body's most important nutrient.

Proteins transport nutrients in and out of cells and carry other materials in the blood. For example, hemoglobin, an iron-carrying protein, carries oxygen from the lungs to all body tissues. The hormone insulin is a protein that regulates the glucose level in blood.

Protein is a component of every cell in the body. Protein makes hair, nails, skin, blood, connective tissue, enzymes, and hormones. A constant supply of protein is needed to repair body cells as they wear out, and to repair injuries. Protein is used to create increased amounts of body tissue needed during periods of growth in infancy, childhood, adolescence, and pregnancy.

Antibodies, manufactured in the body to ward off infectious bacteria and viruses, are proteins. If protein supplies are low, antibody creation is limited, and the body is more susceptible to infection and disease.

AMINO ACIDS: COMPONENTS OF PROTEIN

Protein is composed of numerous amino acids. The body is unable to make some of these amino acids and must obtain them from foods. For this reason, they are termed "essential amino acids." The remainder, which the body can make, are termed "nonessential amino acids." This term is somewhat unfortunate. It does not mean that these amino acids are unimportant, but only that the body can make them.

All of the essential amino acids must be present in a food, and in good proportions, to make a protein food of good quality. Foods of animal origin—eggs, poultry, fish, meat, and dairy products—contain all of the essential amino acids and have high biological values for proteins. Foods of plant origin—grains, nuts, seeds, legumes, fruits, and vegetables—offer other benefits but have protein of lesser value. In foods of plant origin, individual essential amino acids either are too low or lacking. Foods of plant origin have lower biological values than foods of animal origin. For example, histidine, an essential amino acid, is found primarily in animal protein foods. Lysine and threonine, two essential amino acids, are limited in grains. Methionine, an essential amino acid, is limited in beans.

For individuals who eat a mixed diet, an adequate intake of quality protein foods is not difficult to achieve. However, for vegetarians, who shun animal-protein foods, it is difficult to achieve. As the degree of vegetarianism intensifies, with the step-by-step removal of meat, fish, eggs, poultry, and dairy foods from the diet, to the extreme of veganism, the intake of quality protein foods declines and disappears. At the same time, such foods are replaced by large quantities of legumes and grains, foods that are notably lower in quality proteins.

Functions of the Essential Amino Acids

Each essential amino acid has specific functions in the body. Understanding the basic components of protein is important in order to appreciate the vital role of quality proteins.

Histidine

Histidine, discovered as early as 1896, is a precursor of histamine. Histamine is a compound that causes an inflammatory response in the body.

Histidine is important in the production of red and white blood cells. It is a powerful vasodilator and widens blood cells. It is a precursor of hemoglobin. It strengthens the nerve receptors in the inner ear, nourishes the nerve cells of the hearing mechanism, and improves the function of the auditory nerve. Histidine promotes stomach digestive secretions, is an excellent carrier for iron and zinc, and promotes normal sexual response.

Isoleucine

Isoleucine, isolated in 1903, differs from leucine by a methyl group. Isoleucine should always be in well-balanced proportions with two other essential amino acids: leucine and valine.

Isoleucine is the major source of energy for muscles, and is metabolized primarily in muscle tissue. It is essential for the formation of hemoglobin.

Isoleucine reduces stress in the central nervous system, and helps to promote clear thinking. It may be associated with development of the brain and intelligence in the fetus.

Leucine

Leucine was identified as early as 1819, and its chemical structure was established near the end of that century, in 1881. Leucine improves protein synthesis. It needs always to be in well-balanced proportions with two other essential amino acids: valine and isoleucine. Leucine is metabolized in muscle tissue, produces energy in muscle, and readily promotes muscle growth. Also, it stabilizes blood sugar levels. It promotes healing in the skin and of broken bones. It aids in the absorption of another essential amino acid, tryptophan.

Leucine is needed by all species of animals. Signs of leucine deficiency are lack of growth, loss of weight, and negative nitrogen balance, meaning that not enough absorbed nitrogen is retained for growth and maintenance.

Lysine

Lysine was isolated as early as 1899, and its chemical structure was established in 1902. Lysine is one of the first amino acids shown to be necessary for growth in animals. Lysine promotes bone growth by helping to form collagen, the fibrous protein that makes bone, cartilage, and other connective tissues. It aids in calcium absorption, promotes insulin production, improves the uptake of branched-chain amino acids—valine, isoleucine, and leucine—in muscle, increases protein synthesis, and has an antifatigue effect. Lysine produces carnitine (an amino-acid-like substance related to the B vitamins), which improves stress tolerance and fat metabolism. Also, lysine inhibits the growth of viruses and builds antibodies.

Humans who are deficient in lysine may experience nausea, dizziness, and anemia.

Dry heating of protein, such as in the manufacture of ready-to-eat cereals, destroys much of their lysine content, either directly or by irreversible reactions with the carbohydrates in the product.

Methionine

Methionine was isolated in 1922, and its chemical structure was determined in 1928. Methionine is a necessary component of the diet for all animals, including humans. Methionine is required for liver health and the detoxification process. It prevents excessive fat buildup in the liver, and helps to regenerate liver and kidney cells. It reduces estrogen to estradiol (one of the body's main forms of estrogen).

Methionine interacts with other substances in the body to detoxify harmful compounds such as environmental pollutants, radiation, and purines. Purines, compounds produced by some foods, convert to uric acid, which adversely affects gout sufferers. Methionine furnishes sulfur for the biological synthesis of cystine, a nonessential amino acid. Also, methionine is a precursor of choline, betaine, carnitine, creatine, sarcosine, and adrenaline. It is essential for selenium absorption. Methionine promotes antibody production. It also helps prevent premature hair loss.

Phenylalanine

Phenylalanine was isolated as early as 1879. Phenylalanine stimulates the thyroid gland and is used by the gland to make thyroxine (a hormone involved in the regulation of metabolism and heat production) and by the brain to stimulate production of adrenaline and noradrenaline, used by the body to react to stress. Phenylalanine produces neurotransmitters that control impulse transmission between nerve cells, and is involved in dopamine transmission. Dopamine is a neurotransmitter that produces and maintains an elevated and positive mood of alertness and ambition. It enhances learning and memory.

Phenylalanine is a precursor of tyrosine. In sufficient quantities, phenylalanine can eliminate the need for a dietary source of tyrosine, a nonessential amino acid. Phenylalanine metabolism is incomplete in the presence of a vitamin C deficiency.

Phenylketonuria (PKU), a genetic defect, is characterized by a failure to break down phenylalanine. Pregnant women who are PKU carriers must avoid foods containing phenylalanine in order to prevent mental retardation and neurological disorders in their offspring. The condition is treated with phenylalanine-free diets. There is a warning label on aspartame (NutraSweet), the noncaloric sweetener, that it contains phenylalanine and must be avoided by individuals who have this genetic defect.

Threonine

Threonine, isolated in 1935, was the last of the nutritionally important amino acids to be discovered. Threonine is probably necessary for all species of animals, including humans, at all times. Generally, it is low in vegetarian diets. Threonine is essential to normal growth and is an important constituent of collagen and elastin proteins. It improves digestion and food assimilation and aids in the absorption of other nutrients. It prevents fatty buildup in the liver. It strengthens the immune system by producing immunoglobulins and antibodies. It is needed by the thymus (a major gland in the immune system) for T-cell formation and balance. Threonine can be degraded to glycine, a nonessential amino acid.

Tryptophan

Tryptophan was isolated in 1901, and its chemical structure was established in 1907. Tryptophan is used by the brain to produce the neurotransmitter serotonin, which is a mood regulator that can exert a calming effect. It is also a precursor of niacin (vitamin B_3), aiding in the utilization of the vitamin B complex.

Tryptophan stimulates the release of growth hormone, which burns body fat and acts as an aid in weight control. It reduces carbohydrate craving. It promotes growth in smooth muscle.

Valine

Valine was isolated as early as 1856, and its chemical structure was established from 1901 to 1906. Valine is necessary for growth maintenance and nitrogen balance. A deficiency in humans of valine results in an immediate state of nitrogen imbalance. Valine is found mainly in animal-protein foods. This essential amino acid needs always to be in well-balanced proportions with leucine and isoleucine, two other essential amino acids previously discussed.

Valine is a precursor of glycogen (the storage form of glucose) for sustained endurance. The amino acid is metabolized in muscle. It coordinates nerve impulses in muscles and the brain. It sparks mental vigor, muscular coordination, smooth working of the nervous system, promotes restful sleep, and stabilizes emotions and nervousness. Also, it promotes growth hormone release.

Functions of the Nonessential Amino Acids

As mentioned earlier, "nonessential" does not mean that these amino acids are unimportant, but only that the body can make them. The following are nonessential amino acids.

Alanine

Alanine is used as a body fuel by tissues of the brain, nervous system, and muscle. It is important in converting energy to stored energy in the body's Krebs energy cycle. It is glycogenic (glycogen is an energy storage source of glucose by the liver and muscles). Alanine has important nitrogen quality for post-injury states. It strengthens cell walls, builds up the immune system, and produces immunoglobulins and antibodies. It metabolizes sugars and organic acids.

Alanine is essential in the metabolism of tryptophan, an essential amino acid discussed earlier, as well as pyridoxine (vitamin B_6).

Arginine

Arginine is nonessential for children. However, it is vital for optimal growth. It stimulates the release of growth hormone. It is important to muscle metabolism and acts as a vehicle to transport, store, and excrete nitrogen. It increases muscle mass, while decreasing the amount of body fat. By moderating glucose tolerance, arginine helps maintain a good blood sugar level.

Arginine is important in post-injury problems, such as weight changes and maintenance of nitrogen balance. It improves tissue healing.

Arginine increases collagen, the main supportive fibrous protein, as mentioned earlier, that is found in bone, cartilage, and other connective tissues. Also, it stimulates the immune system and combats physical and mental fatigue. It promotes the formation and activation of sperm. It promotes detoxification of ammonia, a byproduct of normal cellular processes that is poisonous to living cells.

Arginine transforms to ornithine, another nonessential amino acid.

Aspartic Acid

Aspartic acid is excitatory, meaning that it increases activity in the central nervous system. Also, it increases the resistance to fatigue. Salts of aspartic acid are involved in energy production and increased stamina and endurance. Aspartic acid is involved in carbohydrate metabolism and nitrogen balance. It protects the liver and promotes normal cell function. It strengthens the immune system and produces immunoglobulins and antibodies.

Aspartic acid is a mineral carrier, especially for magnesium and potassium. Aspartic acid carries these minerals into the mitochondria, which are energy producers for cells.

Aspartic acid works with threonine, an essential amino acid previously discussed.

Citrulline

Citrulline stimulates the immune system and, thereby, benefits any illness, disease, or traumatic injury or wound. Also, it detoxifies ammonia. It helps the body recover from fatigue. Citrulline metabolizes to arginine, another nonessential amino acid just discussed.

Cysteine

Cysteine aggressively scavenges for free radicals and helps prevent damage from the ill effects of cigarette smoke. It detoxifies many other harmful chemicals, such as benzene and cyanide, detoxifies heavy metals, and promotes healing of wounds. Also, it stabilizes carbohydrate metabolism.

Cystine

Cystine is closely related to cysteine, and both readily convert to each other. Like cysteine, cystine aggressively scavenges for free radicals and protects against radiation damage. It contains sulfur, which reacts with other body substances to detoxify harmful compounds.

Cystine stimulates white blood cell activity in the immune system for disease resistance. It promotes recovery from surgery and burns. Like cysteine, it stabilizes carbohydrate metabolism.

Cystine is vital for the formation of skin and hair. Also, it is necessary for utilizing pyridoxine.

Glutamic Acid

Glutamic acid is especially important in brain metabolism. It functions as a brain fuel, serving as an excitatory neurotransmitter. It transports potassium across the blood-brain barrier (a series of semi-permeable partitions that separate and monitor the body and its supply of substances and nutrients to the brain). Glutamic acid combines to form the nonessential amino acid glutamine and, in the process, picks up ammonia radicals. This is the only method that the brain has to detoxify ammonia.

Glutamic acid metabolizes sugars and fats, and it is instrumental in metabolizing other amino acids. It is a component of folic acid and the glucose-tolerance factor.

Glutamine

Like glutamic acid, glutamine is involved with brain metabolism. It, too, is used as a brain fuel. Along with glucose, glutamine is a primary source of energy for the brain. Glutamine sustains mental ability.

Glutamine promotes regeneration of the intestinal mucosa (mucus lining). Also, it reduces the loss of potassium and sodium electrolytes, the form used by most minerals to circulate in the body.

Glycine

Glycine is of special value as a source of creatine, which is essential for muscle function. It breaks down glycogen and frees energy. It builds up the immune system and produces immunoglobulins and antibodies. It inhibits or dampens nerve impulses and calms the brain and nerves.

Glycine is a precursor of serine, another nonessential amino acid. It is an excellent carrier for copper.

The body builds its proteins from an "amino acid pool," and glycine acts as a nitrogen pool to synthesize nonessential amino acids. Glycine completes construction of a protein only after all the required amino acids are present.

Ornithine

Ornithine stimulates the release of growth hormone, which increases muscle mass. It stimulates other hormones, such as insulin. It decreases the amount of body fat. Ornithine strengthens the immune system and promotes healing. It promotes liver function and regeneration. It is important for detoxifying ammonia.

Proline

Proline is extremely important for proper growth and functioning of tendons, joints, joint linings, and good heart muscles. It is a major constituent of collagen and also promotes elasticity of skin. It is an energy storage source of glucose by the liver and muscles. Proline can be converted to the amino acid glutamic acid.

Serine

Along with other nonessential amino acids, serine, too, is an energy storage source of glucose by the liver and muscles. It, too, builds up the immune system and produces immunoglobulins and antibodies. Serine is used to form protective sheaths that surround nerves. It aids in skin metabolism.

Taurine

Although taurine is a nonessential amino acid, it is required for development of the fetal brain and central nervous system. It is vital, too, for the newborn. It is related to brain development. Taurine is one of the most common amino acids in the body, yet it is not found in most foods. The body manufactures it from methionine and cystine, two other nonessential amino acids discussed earlier. Taurine is found in breast milk, one of many benefits bestowed by breastfeeding of the infant.

Taurine is found in high concentrations in the tissues of the heart, the skeletal muscle, and the central nervous system. It calms neurotransmitters, moderates cholesterol production and fat metabolism, improves digestion, and improves disorders of the ileum (the end of the small intestine). It is a precursor of bile. Taurine prevents cardiac loss of potassium and binds calcium.

Tyrosine

Tyrosine is the precursor of thyroid and adrenal hormones. Tyrosine plays important roles in the functioning of the adrenal, pituitary, and thyroid glands.

Tyrosine is a brain stimulant and elevates mood. It produces melanin and is responsible for pigmentation of the skin and hair. Tyrosine stimulates the release of growth hormone, which causes muscle growth and reduces body fat. Tyrosine generates red and white blood cells.

MEASURING PROTEIN QUALITY IN FOOD

There are several methods of measuring protein quality in food. All measurements demonstrate clearly that foods from animal sources have better protein quality than those from plant sources.

One method measures the "biological values" of foods. This term denotes the percentage of absorbed nitrogen retained for growth and maintenance. A sampling of whole foods is listed on the next page in the descending order of their biological values (measured in milligrams per 100 grams of food).

Another method is the protein efficiency ratio (PER). The quality of protein is measured by the protein's ability to support growth in young rats. Findings are similar to those of biological values. The protein in animal foods containing all the essential amino acids is better than the protein in plant foods, which are low or lacking in some essential amino acids.

Food	Biological Value (mg/g)	Food	Biological Value (mg/g)
Whole human milk	95	Whole wheat	67
Whole egg	94	White potato	67
Whole cow's milk	90	Whole oat	66
Egg albumin (white)	83	Whole barley	64
Animal liver	77	Whole corn	60
Beef	76	Whole rye	58
Fish	76	Peanut	56
Brown rice	75	Peas/beans	40

The PER method has been replaced by another, known as protein digestibility-corrected amino acid scoring (PDCAAS). This newer method presumably depicts protein quality more accurately, because it is based on the needs of humans rather than young rats. Also, PDCAAS balances the value of plant proteins with that of animal proteins.

A protein's PDCAAS score is calculated by analyzing the essential amino acid (levels in milligrams per gram of protein) with an analytical testing method. Then, a determination is made of the uncorrected amino acid score for each of the essential amino acids by dividing the milligrams of essential amino acid in 1 gram of test protein (the value having been derived from the analytical testing procedure) by the milligrams of essential amino acid in 1 gram of reference protein established by the Food & Agriculture Organization (FAO) and the World Health Organization (WHO). Finally, multiplying the lowest of the uncorrected amino acid scores by the food's true digestibility value, the PDCAAS score is achieved. A "perfect score" is 1.00. Proteins with this value provide all essential amino acids and are considered to be complete protein sources. Although *excess* amino acids are broken down and utilized by the body, generally they are not used for protein synthesis. Casein (from milk) and albumin (egg white) possess scores of 1.00; kidney beans, 0.68; and whole wheat, 0.40.

Once more, it is demonstrated that foods from animal sources have higher protein quality than foods from plant sources. This feature has health implications for everyone. It brings into question the unsound official recommendations weighted heavily in favor of plant foods. Both the USDA Food Guide Pyramid and official pronouncements encourage more plant-food consumption at the expense of quality protein foods. Also, we are told that we are consuming adequate, or perhaps too much, protein. This statement, too, may be an unsound judgment.

The 2005 revised Food Guide Pyramid denigrates quality protein foods. Foods from animal protein are combined with beans into one category, without distinguishing differences in protein quality of the two. The Pyramid recommends the number of ounces of protein foods that should be consumed daily: 6 ounces for men; 5, for women; and 3 to 4, for children. The revised Pyramid repeats the fallacious recommendation of past Pyramids. Among many shortcomings, the current Pyramid continues to make no distinction between proteins of high or low quality. Actually, it discourages the use of high-quality protein by its recommendation to use foods low in saturated fat and cholesterol. This recommendation targets foods from animal sources. On the other hand, the Pyramid encourages the use of low-fat foods, which are imbalanced foods. It encourages the use of polyunsaturated oils, which are health-damaging oils. Apparently, in formulating the new Pyramid, as with the previous Pyramids, decisions were made based on industry lobby pressures rather than scientific findings.

RE-EXAMINING PROTEIN REQUIREMENTS

According to the National Research Council, which establishes the U.S. Recommended Dietary Allowances (RDAs), there is "little evidence that muscular activity increases the need for protein." The WHO stated that "energy requirements change with activity and lifestyle [but] protein requirements do not." However, both organizations based their daily protein recommendation primarily on studies of sedentary men and women. Yet more and more Americans now engage in regular exercise and probably require more protein.

The current RDA, which suggests 0.89 grams (g) of protein per kilogram (kg) of body weight per day for adults of all ages, may not meet the needs of the elderly. A growing body of evidence from scientific studies suggests that the nutrient needs of the elderly may be greater than those of young adults. Most of the studies indicate that a protein intake of 1.0 g or more per kg is likely to be the amount to meet an elderly person's needs. A review of the data currently available indicates that approximately 50 percent of free-living elderly people and 25 percent of the institutionalized elderly habitually consume less than this amount of protein. The researchers suggested that future editions of the RDAs should base protein allowances for the elderly on studies conducted among people in that age group, rather than extrapolating from studies conducted in younger people. (*Nutrition Today*, September/October 1996; 13: 192–197)

Another study, conducted by Carmen Castaneda, M.D., Ph.D., and Marilyn C. Crim at the USDA's Jean Mayer Human Nutrition Research Center on Aging at Tufts University found that older women developed health problems when their intake of protein was low. They had a significant drop in lean body mass, muscle function, and the ability to ward off infection. For a 140-pound woman, the RDA is 50 grams a day. While most Americans may meet or exceed this level, some 10 to 20 percent of women over fifty-five years of age eat less than 30 grams a day. The researchers wanted to see if such a low protein intake would compromise women's immune response, as well as their ability to be mobile and perform normal tasks, even if the women had a sufficient intake of calories.

Six volunteer women, all over sixty-six years of age, ate about half the RDA for protein for nine weeks. Six others of the same age group ate a little more protein than the RDA level. The women eating only half the protein of the RDA lost an average 8 percent of lean tissue, most of which was muscle. A hypersensitivity skin test—a measure of immune response—was 50 percent lower by the end of the study. The amount of weight they could push in a chest-press exercise dropped by 12 percent. In contrast, the women eating ample amounts of protein showed no changes in muscle mass. Moreover, several measurements of their muscle function and immune response improved significantly, as did several blood-protein measurements. The findings with this group suggest that their diet, prior to the study, may have been slightly low in meeting their protein needs.

Another study at Tufts University, conducted six years later in 2001, suggested that protein may be important in reducing bone loss in the elderly. The seventy-to-ninety-year-old men and women in the highest protein-intake group lost significantly less bone over a four-year period than those in the group with a protein intake only half as much, or less. Animal protein, as well as overall protein intake, was associated with the prevention of bone loss.

This finding runs counter to studies of younger people with diets high in protein, especially animal protein that caused the body to excrete more calcium. However, the finding confirms several large-population studies showing protein to have an overall positive effect on bone. (*Journal of Bone and Mineral Research*, 2000; 15: 2504–2512)

Other groups of people also may benefit from higher protein intake. The Nurses' Health Study, discussed earlier, showed that women consuming the most protein—eating some 24 percent of their calories from protein daily—lowered their risk of heart disease. They had only 75 percent as much risk as the women who ate only 15 percent of their calories from protein daily. The conventional wisdom, favoring plant protein over animal protein to reduce heart disease risk, may be flawed. The Nurses' Health Study showed that animal protein appeared as protective as plant protein. (*American Journal of Clinical Nutrition*, Aug 1999)

Elsewhere, the risk of heart disease was studied in relation to low- and high-protein diets. Bernard M. Wolfe, M.D., who led the study at the University of Western Ontario, Canada, switched men and women at high risk of heart disease between diets low or high in protein. During the high-protein phase, the participants' blood concentrations of triglycerides and low-density lipoprotein (LDL) cholesterol levels (considered unfavorable) fell, and their high-density lipoprotein (HDL) cholesterol levels (considered favorable) rose. All three of these changes are thought to be beneficial in reducing heart disease risk. A follow-up study with healthy people showed similar but smaller benefits of proteins in reducing heart disease risk.

The common recommendation to eat more carbohydrate and less protein in order to reduce heart disease risk is advice that may be toppled. In an Australian study, vegetarians and meat eaters volunteered in a study of heart disease risk. Of 139 healthy male participants, aged twenty to fifty-five years, 18 were vegans (persons eating no animal foods or byproducts); 43, lacto-ovovegetarians (persons eating dairy products and eggs, but not meat or fish); 60 moderate meat eaters; and 18 high-meat eaters. The two meat-eating groups consumed significantly greater amounts of methionine than vegetarians. Methionine is low or lacking in soybeans and in other plant foods used by vegetarians. As discussed earlier, methionine is an essential amino acid. In the participants, the plasma concentrations of vitamin B_{12} (cyanocobalamin) decreased progressively from the high-meat eaters to the vegans. The meat eaters showed the lowest amount of fasting plasma homocysteine concentrations; the vegans, the highest. Homocysteine is a marker for heart disease risk; the higher the homocysteine level, the greater is the risk. Homocysteine can be lowered by including vitamin B_{12} (as well as B_6 and folates) in the diet. Unless vegetarians use a B_{12} supplement, their diets provide little, if any, B_{12}; the vegan diet provides no B_{12}. The increased homocysteine concentrations in the vegetarian diets may indicate an increased risk of heart attack. (*European Journal of Clinical Nutrition*, 1999; 53: 895–899)

Another study, led by Bernard M. Wolfe and L. A. Piche, suggests that replacing some carbohydrate in the diet with high-protein food can result in an improved plasma lipid (fat) profile in healthy adults. Ten healthy volunteers with normal lipid levels were fed either a low- or high-protein diet, with equal amounts of calories, for four weeks. The low-protein diet had 12 percent protein; the high-protein diet, 22 percent.

After eating the diets for the full term of the experiment, the participants on the high-protein diet showed lower values for mean plasma cholesterol concentrations than those on the low-protein diet. The high-protein diet led to plasma total cholesterol that was 7 percent lower; LDL cholesterol, 8 percent lower; VLDL (very-low-density lipoprotein) cholesterol, 23 percent lower; TAG (triacylglycerol, a triglyceride), 27 percent lower; and total cholesterol to HDL cholesterol ratio, 11 percent lower. The HDL cholesterol was slightly higher (4 percent) after following the high-protein diet, and the subjects from this group reported feeling slightly more satiated in following the high-protein diet. The study demonstrated that when carbohydrate is replaced with a higher amount of protein in the diet, but with no change in the percent of fat calories, it leads to an improved plasma lipid and lipoprotein profile in adults with normal cholesterol levels. (See *Clinical Investigative Medicine*, 1999, vol. 22, pp. 140–148.) Similar results had been demonstrated earlier in postmenopausal women with high cholesterol levels.

SELECTING QUALITY PROTEIN FOODS

Quality protein foods contain all the essential amino acids, and the amino acids are in a good state of balance. Quality protein foods are derived from animal, not plant, sources.

Eggs

The egg is the germ of animal life, as the seed is the germ of plant life. The egg is one of the most nutritious and balanced foods. It contains all of the essential and nonessential amino acids, as well as many vitamins, minerals, and trace minerals, and the various components are in good ratios to one another.

Despite the excellent values of the egg, during the 1970s, this food was maligned wrongfully due to the misguided concern about cholesterol. The scare led to official recommendations to limit egg consumption, and to numerous attempts to reduce, or even eliminate, the cholesterol content in the egg.

Ultimately, the emphasis shifted. Researchers at the University of Arizona in Tucson conducted a meta-analysis of more than thirty years of research and concluded that "for most healthy people, the cholesterol they eat does not raise their cholesterol levels. Healthy individuals with normal cholesterol levels should now feel free to enjoy foods like eggs in their diet every day," reported Wanda Howell, Ph.D., R.D., spokesperson for the researchers, quoted in *Prepared Foods* (June 1998). The meta-analysis study was published in the June 1997 issue of the *American Journal of Clinical Nutrition.*

After this finding and others, efforts shifted toward improving the egg's nutritional quality. By then, research findings were showing that the quality of fat in the egg was important, with increasing emphasis on the benefits of omega-3 fatty acids. The search began for sources of omega-3 that would be suitable for use in the feed of laying hens.

At Texas University, poultry researchers fortified the diet of laying hens with fish oil, rich in omega-3, to yield egg yolks higher in these fatty acids. However, the fish oil used from menhaden (a herringlike ocean fish regarded as a "trash" fish only suitable for pet food) proved to be too "fishy" a taste in the eggs.

Marine algae were substituted to produce "nutritionally enhanced" eggs. An added benefit was an intense yolk color, provided by the pigment present in the algae.

At the University of Arizona, researchers substituted chia seeds, rich in plant-derived omega-3 fatty acids, to constitute 12 percent of the fat in the eggs. The ratio of saturated to polyunsaturated fats in these eggs was half that in ordinary eggs. Also, the chia bestowed a longer shelf life to the eggs.

Purslane was also considered. This weedy herb is the richest known source of omega-3 fatty acids in leafy green plants. Purslane was investigated by Norman Salem, Jr., Ph.D., a lipid biochemist at the National Institutes of Health, with Artemis P. Simopoulos, M.D., at the American Association for World Health.

The researchers found that the yolks from large eggs produced on a Greek farm by free-range hens feeding on purslane contained about 300 mg of omega-3 fatty acids. This was the equivalent omega-3 content of standard fish-oil capsules and ten times the amount that is found in a typical American supermarket egg.

Another source of omega-3 fatty acids considered by Texas A&M University researchers was flaxseed oil. More than half of the oil in the flaxseed consists of alpha-linolenic acid, an omega-3 fatty acid. Some alpha-linolenic acid is changed in the human body into two substances: EPA (eicosapentaenoic acid) and DHA (docosahexaenoic acid). These substances are found in fish, too, and are thought to be beneficial to health, especially in helping to prevent heart disease.

As a result of the flaxseed research, a Texas-based egg producer began to sell eggs from hens given feed fortified with flaxseed and vitamin E. The eggs had about as much saturated and monounsaturated fats as ordinary eggs. However, they contained 10 milligrams each of alpha-linolenic acid and DHA, and ten times as much vitamin E as found in ordinary eggs.

Although fish oil had proved too "fishy" for the feed of laying hens, other foods from the sea, such as marine algae and kelp (seaweed) were examined. Marine algae added to the feed produced eggs high in DHA. Unfortunately, kelp had a drawback. The FDA decided that the iodine content in the feed from the seaweed was at a level sufficiently high to make the eggs a health hazard. The FDA ordered a halt to the sale of eggs from hens fed kelp. The sellers reformulated the feed so that the iodine level in the eggs would be well below the RDA, and at an amount that the FDA would deem safe and appropriate.

In Japan, vitamin D–fortified dried shiitake mushroom powder was added, experimentally, to the feed of hens, to produce vitamin D–fortified eggs. The vitamin D content in the egg yolk was increased about ten times, compared to ordinary eggs.

In Finland, at the Agricultural Research Center, the vitamin D content of eggs was raised sevenfold by tripling the vitamin D in the feed of laying hens. One egg daily would provide enough for the official recommendation for vitamin D intake.

As a result of these various attempts to improve the nutritional offerings in eggs, some cartons now sold are labeled as being high in omega-3 fatty acids. If they are available, the eggs are superior to ordinary commercially produced ones. However, they are pricey. Some of these eggs are packaged in look-through plastics that have been chosen, no doubt, to appeal to shoppers. If you purchase eggs in such containers, transfer them to old-fashioned cardboard cartons that are safer as storage containers than plastics.

The safety of polystyrene egg containers—shiny satin pastels in appearance—were investigated by the Louisiana Agricultural Experiment Station in 1991. The researchers reported that volatile styrene monomers were detected in shell eggs stored in the containers for two weeks in supermarkets. Egg dishes cooked with these contaminated eggs contained seven times more ethylbenzene and styrene than those prepared from fresh farm eggs that had not been packaged in polystyrene. It was suspected that the volatile compounds can migrate through the porous shells into the edible portions of the eggs. (*Journal of Food Science*, Mar/Apr 1991)

Shop for eggs that have been produced from free-range hens, fed no growth hormones, antibiotics, or medications. The hens should be raised in farm environments where pesticides are not applied. These facts may be stated on egg cartons. Seek certified organic or biodynamic eggs, if they are available. You may also wish to look for cartons labeled "free farmed." This program, launched by the American Humane Society, informs consumers that eggs (as well as meat and dairy products) have been produced by animals "humanely raised." The program is intended to increase public awareness of farm-animal treatment and to serve as a national standard to improve farm conditions. Farmers who display the "free farmed" food label must meet a set of standards for housing, feeding, and the environment, created by a team of experts in animal care and checked by the USDA.

Cartons of eggs should be refrigerated in grocery stores, and the cartons should be dated. Check that the eggs in the carton are sound and not cracked or leaking. Unsound eggs can admit bacteria and other unwanted contaminants.

Eggs have a relatively long shelf life in the home refrigerator. After several weeks, they are still safe to eat, but their quality begins to decline. After shelling, the yolk of a fresh egg stands up; a stale one flattens out.

Keep eggs in their original cardboard container. Do not transfer them to egg slots that are in some refrigerator doors. That area is not as cold as the interior of the refrigerator. Also, open to the air, the eggs can absorb odors and tastes from other stored foods.

Do not consume raw or undercooked eggs. There is a risk of salmonella poisoning, especially from the virulent strain, *S. enteritidis.* Do not eat commercially prepared foods that contain raw or undercooked eggs, such as Caesar salad, eggnog, or meringue.

Due to the potential for *S. enteritidis* to contaminate pooled eggs used in restaurants, nursing homes, and other institutions of mass feeding, some eggs are sold that already have been pasteurized. It is not necessary for the ordinary shopper to purchase such eggs, because pasteurization is achieved at home when eggs are cooked properly.

Gentle heat is best to retain nutrients when eggs are poached, shirred, coddled, or soft- or hard-cooked. A greenish ring around hard-cooked eggs indicates that they have been cooked too long. Stir-frying or sautéing is preferable to hard frying with high heat. The whites of the eggs should turn from being translucent to opaque in cooking.

There are many myths about eggs that need to be dispelled. Here is a sampling:

Myth 1: "Brown-shell eggs cost more than white-shell eggs because they are better." Wrong. Brown-shell eggs are more expensive to produce. The hens are larger and therefore consume more feed. Relative to demand for brown-shell eggs, the supply is small. Less than 10 percent of all eggs produced nationally are brown shell. Some consumers are willing to pay the higher price—about 10 percent more—because they regard brown-shell eggs as more "natural" or "countrylike." The brown shells may be slightly stronger than white shells. They are more impervious to light, which makes it harder to see cracks or blood spots in them during handling operations. However, there is no nutritional difference between brown- and white-shell eggs. Both types are nourishing.

Myth 2: "For safety, wash eggs before refrigerating them." Wrong. The USDA advises consumers not to wash eggs before refrigerating them. Washing would remove the protective coating applied to the shell eggs at the packing plant.

Myth 3: "For health reasons, one should eat egg whites, but limit consumption of yolks." Wrong. Both are healthy. The yolk contains all of the egg's nutritious fats and many of its vitamins. A, D, and E, being fat-soluble vitamins, are solely in the yolk, and about half of the total protein is in the yolk. Also, the yolk contains all of the zinc, and more phosphorus, manganese, iron, iodine, copper, and calcium than is found in the white. The egg white is mostly protein—of high biological value—and some carbohydrate. Also, the white contains riboflavin (vitamin B_2), niacin, choline, folate, magnesium, potassium, sodium, sulfur, and vitamin B_{12}. Obviously, for optimal nutrition, the egg should be eaten with both the yolk and white together. It serves as a reminder that *whole foods are more nutritious and balanced than partitioned ones.*

Myth 4: "One should limit egg consumption to no more than three or four a week." This recommendation is baseless. For good health, and especially for heart health, one can eat eggs freely. The folly of egg restriction has been demonstrated repeatedly. One study, at Kansas State University, published in the *Journal of Nutrition* in 2001, showed that cholesterol absorption from eggs is reduced by lecithin, a substance also present in eggs. Lecithin, a type of fatty acid, interferes with the uptake of cholesterol in the human intestines. The researchers concluded that most people should not be concerned about eating *one or two eggs daily.*

The late Roger J. Williams, Ph.D., an eminent nutritional researcher, noted years ago that eggs are beneficial to general health and the cardiovascular system, too. By excluding cholesterol-containing foods such as eggs, the body manufactures even more cholesterol.

Low-cholesterol egg substitutes, consisting of egg whites and chemicals to replace the yolks, were introduced in the mid-1970s. More money was spent on advertisements than research with these products. After the products were launched, nutritional researchers M. K. Navidi and F. A. Kummerow, at the University of Illinois at Urbana, attempted to learn whether these products met the growth requirement of weanling rats.

In laboratory experiments, Navidi and Kummerow fed one group of rats (the control) a standard stock diet; another group was fed Egg Beaters; and a third group was fed whole farm-fresh eggs. At three weeks of age, pups from the mother rats fed the standard stock diet weighed an average of 70 grams; those on Egg Beaters, only 31.6 grams; and those on whole eggs, 66.5 grams. Both the mothers and pups fed Egg Beaters developed diarrhea within a week of feeding; those on whole eggs did not. The general appearance of the rats on Egg Beaters indicated "a gross deficiency in one or more nutritional factors" compared to those fed whole eggs or the stock diet. The researchers concluded that "it is evident that shell eggs, which contain egg yolk, furnish one or more nutritional factors which are absent in Egg Beaters. These nutritional factors are no doubt present in the common food items that comprise the diet of human adults [but] may not be present in adequate amounts for infants fed milk and Egg Beaters instead of egg yolk from a soft-boiled egg." The pups fed the eggs were weaned at five weeks of age and were healthy. *All of the pups fed the egg substitute died within three to four weeks after weaning.* (*Pediatrics*, Apr 1974; also the *Journal of Food Science*, Jan/Feb 1975)

Navidi and Kummerow concurred with the recommendations of the Council of the American Medical Association, which had stated, "Care [must] be taken to assure that the dietary advice given does not compromise the intake of essential nutrients." The Council recommended that no drastic dietary changes be made; it considered as unwise any action to remove cholesterol from infant foods, curtail the amount of eggs, meat, and dairy products consumed by growing children, replace such foods with polyunsaturated oils, and so forth. Any such radical dietary changes might, in the opinion of the Council, "result in nutritional disaster."

Another animal-feeding experiment reinforced the findings of Navidi and Kummerow. Using white leghorn chicks, researchers compared several commonly used food products, including egg substitutes, breakfast cereals, and doughnuts, to hard-cooked eggs and starter mash, formulated as a balanced mix for young chicks. Each food was fed to the chicks for three weeks. Then, all chicks were shifted to a starter mash. Chicks receiving the Egg Beaters lost weight, and *all of the animals in this group were dead within twelve days after the trial began.* The only groups without mortality were those chicks on hard-cooked eggs and on the starter-mash diet. Experiments such as this are criticized because the animals were fed single food items. However, the researchers justified the experiment: "It is obvious that one does not consume a single food. However, single food feeding dramatically demonstrates biological differences better than comparing them in food analysis tables." (*Poultry Times*, 25 Mar 1975)

Myth 5: "Cholesterol-containing foods, such as eggs, are bad for health." Wrong. Despite popular misconceptions, cholesterol is a useful substance and essential in the body. Cholesterol is necessary for many processes. It affects the production of steroid hormones and bile acids. It serves as a structural component of cellular membranes.

After clearing up some misconceptions about eggs, it is necessary, however, to state that eggs are not for everyone. Eggs can be allergenic for some individuals. For them, label reading is essential. "Albumin" may not be a familiar term on a label. It signifies that the food product contains an egg component (egg white). Also, some vaccines contain egg. The egg-allergic individual needs to be vigilant.

For the vast majority of people who are egg tolerant, this food is a good choice. For the shopper, the egg usually is the least costly of all quality protein foods. Following the wise dictum of eating as wide a variety of basic foods as possible, try eggs from fowl other than chickens. If you have the opportunity, eat eggs from ducks, geese, turkeys, quails, or even ostriches.

Poultry

Much of what has been discussed above about selecting quality eggs also applies to selecting quality poultry. The fowl should be free-range, and fed non-medicated quality feed. Look for the USDA organic seal on poultry. If available, buy locally raised birds that are fresh and have never been frozen.

Rather than purchasing chickens in parts, select a whole bird and ask the butcher to quarter it. After cooking the parts, some can be consumed immediately and the rest frozen for future use. Add livers and necks to soups.

If you plan to debone the cooked chickens, save the bones. Place them in a saucepan, cover them with water or vegetable juices, add a little vinegar to extract valuable minerals from the bones, and simmer. Cool and strain. This broth is a good addition to soups and stews.

Older birds (hens) are less costly than younger birds (broilers). The older birds require moist cooking, as with soups and stews.

As with eggs, there are some common misconceptions about poultry. Here are a few:

Myth 1: "Wash raw chicken before cooking it." This is poor advice, according to Susan Templin Conley, a USDA staff member on its Meat and Poultry Hotline. Most likely, raw poultry is contaminated with pathogens. By washing the bird, some of the pathogens contaminate your hands and the sink. Running water will not rid the bird totally of pathogens, but thorough cooking will deactivate all of them. The safest practice is to handle raw poultry minimally. Discard the packaging wrap carefully, and wash your hands thoroughly in hot soapy water after handling raw poultry or other raw animal foods. If you have used a cutting board, sanitize the board and the cutting knife.

Myth 2: "To lower one's fat intake, remove the skin and any fat pads under the skin of poultry before cooking it." No. By doing so, the cooked poultry will be dry and unappetizing. By following this foolhardy procedure, a person may resort to coating the poultry with some vegetable oil, and end up with no reduction of fat—and possibly have even more fat! Also, do not follow the common suggestion to discard cooked chicken skin and fat. Both are healthful, provided they come from well-raised poultry.

Myth 3: "Yellow-hued chickens have more fat than paler birds." Not necessarily. The yellow coloring may come from the pigment in the bird's feed. Formerly, it was achieved by feeding corn to chicken. However, corn has been replaced by other less costly feed that also contains the same yellow pigment (xanthophyll). According to the National Broiler Council, consumers in the Northeast prefer yellow-hued chickens, and Southerners prefer paler birds. Contrary to popular belief, the chicken skin is not a measure of fat content, or of nutritional value, flavor, or tenderness in young chickens.

Myth 4: "On turkey labels, the phrase 'fresh' is reliable." Not necessarily. In 1997, the USDA decided that any fowl stored below 0°F is "frozen," but if the fowl is stored above 26°F it can be considered "fresh." However, at this temperature, the bird is neither frozen nor fresh. This murky determination allows producers to freeze turkeys, ship them interstate for long distances, and sell them at premium prices as "fresh." An alternative phrase, "hard chilled" was suggested, but rejected.

Myth 5: "It is just as safe to cook a turkey in a microwave as in a traditional oven." No. A microwave oven frequently cooks food unevenly, and this is especially hazardous for a large bird such as a turkey, or a meat roast. The result is that a large mass, such as a turkey, may have undercooked portions where viable pathogens are lodged. For the same reason, it is prudent to cook any stuffing in an oven dish, rather than in the bird's cavity, whether one is cooking in a microwave or a conventional oven. Stuffing may not cook evenly in the bird's interior, regardless of the type of oven.

For safety questions regarding poultry, call the USDA's Meat and Poultry Hotline (888-674-6854, or fax 202-690-3754 or 3755, or e-mail mphotline. fsis@usda.gov). Questions are answered by home economists, dietitians, and food technologists. In addition, timely recorded messages are available twenty-four hours a day by using a telephone "menu" at the website www. usda.gov/fsis.

Whenever you have an opportunity to vary your intake of fowl, eat squab, quail, turkey, duck, or goose, in addition to chicken. If you have access, do try wild fowl such as mud hen, partridge, pheasant, guinea hen, wild duck, or turkey.

Fish

Our grandparents may have coaxed us to eat the fish placed before us because it was "brain food." Although this description sounds like a proverbial old wives' tale, there is a modicum of truth in the description. Fish, especially from the sea, contains many minerals and trace minerals that nourish the brain, as well as other parts of the body. In addition, fish has other attributes. It is a quality protein food. Fatty fish species, such as salmon, mackerel, and herring, contain highly beneficial omega-3 fatty acids. There is a far greater variety of quality protein foods from fish than from land animals, especially if one depends on domesticated animals. Such variety with fish is especially helpful for anyone who follows a rotation diet to prevent or lessen food allergies. (On a rotation diet, any one food is not repeatedly eaten for several days. In cases of severe allergic reactions, foods may not be repeated for longer periods of time.)

Unfortunately, fish variety has dwindled for several reasons. As fish farming has developed, only a few species have been chosen. They are mainly salmon, catfish, trout, tilapia, and shrimp. As wild fish have been overfished and have declined in numbers, fewer species are available. Among them, some have become so alarmingly decimated (an example is cod) that even when these species are available, consumers concerned about environmental degradation should not purchase them.

Fish farming has come into existence under the pretense of being an alternative to wild fish. Unfortunately, it is an undesirable alternative and should be regarded as an extension of industrialized land farming; it is organized similarly, and results in similar problems. Fish farming is intensive rearing and requires a range of medications to control illnesses. Fish farming feeds the confined fish uneconomically. According to Rosamond L. Naylor, Ph.D., an agricultural economist at Stanford University's Center for Environmental Science and Policy, about 2.4 pounds of wild fish are required to produce 1 pound of farmed salmon. Salmon, being carnivores, must be fed fish to remain healthy and grow normally. This depletes the ocean's stock of sardines, anchovies, mackerel, herring, and other fish, which are used to produce the compressed pellets fed to farmed salmon. Thus, the strain is not taken off wild fisheries, but rather, it is compounded.

Farmed fish creates additional problems. They create pollution. Their waste, as well as their uneaten food, smother the sea floor beneath the fish farms and generate bacteria that consume oxygen vital to shellfish and other bottom-dwelling sea creatures. Farmed fish, escaping from pens or cages, overwhelm and decimate wild fish. Fish farming, presumed to help alleviate the depletion of marine life from overfishing, actually aggravates the problem.

Farmed salmon, which is especially popular, has a lower level of omega-3 fatty acids—the very constituent that makes salmon so attractive to health-minded shoppers. Nor is farmed salmon as flavorsome as wild salmon. It is comparable to the difference between a domesticated Long Island duckling and a wild duck. The color of farmed salmon would be pale and unappealing were it not for the pigment added to its feed to approximate the color of wild salmon.

Due to marine environmental degradation, all fish, both wild and farmed, now show alarming levels of numerous toxins, including PCBs (polychlorinated biphenyls), dioxins, mercury, and other heavy metals. However, levels of these substances appear to be lower in wild fish than in farmed ones. Also, the level depends on where the fish is caught. Some regions of the world are less polluted than other areas. For example, presently the waters surrounding Iceland are *relatively* clean, and frozen Icelandic fish is esteemed.

Although fresh fish is desirable, fast-frozen fish from a relatively unpolluted area may be a better choice than fresh fish from a heavily polluted area. Large fishing boats carry equipment to freeze fish promptly on board, rather than to store them with ice until the voyage ends.

Certain fish species show high levels of mercury. Among them are swordfish, fresh tuna, and tilefish. The FDA as well as local health authorities have issued warnings that mercury-accumulating fish should be consumed in limited quantities, if at all, and pregnant women should avoid them completely.

At the fish market or fish counter, ask if the fish is farmed or wild. As more people ask this question, the likelihood is greater that information will become available.

If you plan to purchase fresh whole fish, look for signs of freshness. The skin or scales of finfish should glisten and the eyes should be bright. Signs of deterioration are slimy skins and eye opacities. Fresh fish should not have any strong "fishy" smell, which denotes deterioration.

At restaurants, inquire if the fish is farmed or wild. Some upscale restaurants state this information on menus, as well as information about the point of origin of the fish. Do not be misled by the term "Atlantic salmon." Such fish may come originally from stock of the Atlantic species, but are farmed on the Pacific coast! Choose cold-water ocean fish such as salmon, mackerel, and herring. Such fish contribute omega-3 fatty acids in abundance.

Avoid lake fish. Such fish are apt to be more contaminated because the water basin is a contained body with no entry or exit of water. Toxins may keep accumulating to higher and higher levels within the contained basin.

Select small fish rather than large ones. The longer the creature lives, the greater is the toxin bioaccumulation.

If you engage in sports fishing, in dressing caught fish, discard the skin, fat pads, and innards in order to minimize the toxins consumed. Fish only in safe waters.

After handling raw fish, follow the same safety practices with wrappings, cutting board, implements, and hand washing as previously described for poultry.

Avoid eating raw or undercooked fish, such as oysters, clams, herring, sushi, ceviche, or sashimi. Raw finfish and shellfish frequently contain live bacteria, viruses, or parasites. Everyone is at risk, but especially people with liver disease or impaired immune systems. Cook all fish adequately to kill pathogens.

Milk, Cheeses, and Cultured-Milk Products

Milk has been termed "a special fluid," and so it is. Breast milk nurtures the human infant, and the milk from other mammals sustains their offspring.

Milk is a quality protein food, as well as a good source of minerals, trace minerals, vitamins, fats, and other nutrients. Unfortunately, as a result of the industrialization of the food supply, milk has undergone radical transformation. Fresh milk, formerly produced from grass-grazing animals, presently is ultra-pasteurized, homogenized, irradiated with synthetic vitamin D, and fat reduced. It may contain residues of medications and agricultural toxins.

The misguided official recommendation to reduce fat in the diet has led to the craze for fat-reduced and nonfat milk. The late Henry A. Schroeder, M.D., a recognized authority on trace minerals, lamented over the folly of such partitioning of whole foods. Schroeder noted that with removal of fat from whole milk, vanadium, chromium, manganese, cobalt, nickel, copper, and selenium are lost. The rest of the milk retains magnesium, molybdenum, and zinc. This partitioning creates nutrient losses and imbalances, and destroys vital relationships. For example, the milk fat needs to be combined with the magnesium for proper metabolism. This example of food partitioning illustrates the truism that whole foods offer better nutrition than fractured ones.

Milk fat should be consumed. It contains a valuable constituent, conjugated linoleic acid (CLA). This fatty acid is found in many foods of animal origin. It was identified as recently as the mid-1980s in hamburger meat. Foods highest in CLA are full-fat dairy products such as whole milk, whole-milk yogurt, whole-fat cheeses, cream, and butter; and meats such as beef, lamb, and goat. Other foods that contain some CLA, at lower levels, are poultry, pork, and fish. CLA is produced by bacteria in the animal's rumen.

CLA has been found capable of slowing the progress of heart disease and some types of cancer. Despite being a fat component, CLA appears to reduce body fat and its storage, decrease fat-cell size and production, and increase fat burning. High amounts of CLA in the diet also may help fight cachexia, a wasting disease that compromises the survival of many individuals, such as those with malaria or cancer.

Formerly, CLA was abundant in the American diet. However, changes in agricultural practices have reduced its availability drastically. The amount of CLA present in foods from animal sources depends on the quality of their feed. Tilak Dhiman, Ph.D., and his colleagues at Utah State University found that the CLA content of cow's milk was as much as five times higher when cows grazed on green pastures rather than feed mixtures with hay.

With changes to animal feeding practices in industrial agriculture, human access to CLA in food has declined. Dhiman noted that, formerly, animals grazed mainly in pastures. Now, their controlled rations impact negatively on human health. Currently, we produce milk more efficiently, but this should be accompanied by milk quality, achieved in part by the presence of CLA.

CLA intake by many Americans has been lowered still further due to dietary choices. The current craze for low- and no-fat foods, and the popularity of the extreme form of vegetarianism (veganism) in which all foods from animal origin are shunned, have led to a deficiency of CLA among many Americans.

Identification of CLA and studies regarding its benefits challenge the wisdom of official recommendations to select low-fat and no-fat food products. Such advice lacks a scientific basis. At the same time, the findings about the benefits of CLA suggest some value of full-fat dairy foods. Many low- and no-fat food products are not low in calories, due to the increased use of sugars in such products. CLA is a component of the fat in dairy foods. If the fat is reduced or eliminated, access to the benefits of CLA is lessened or depleted.

Yogurt, Kefir, and Other Cultured-Milk Products

Yogurt, kefir, and other cultured-milk products are beneficial foods. They contain all of the nutrients present in fresh fluid milk from which they are made, and the levels of some nutrients actually increase when the milk is fermented. For example, the biological value of protein increases. Some vitamins, notably fractions of the vitamin B complex, are synthesized by bacteria in the fermented milk, as well as by bacteria present in the human intestinal tract. For example, the intestinal flora synthesize pyridoxine and allow tryptophan to form niacin (another vitamin B fraction). The levels of folic and folinic acids (also vitamin B fractions) increase in milk through fermentation.

The probiotic qualities of cultured-milk products are well established. As early as 1899, bifidobacteria were identified in fermented milk at the Pasteur Institute in Paris. Subsequent research has continued to add knowledge about the benefits of probiotic bacteria.

Cultured-milk products develop powerful lactic-acid bacteria that hinder the growth of, or kill outright, some virulent pathogenic organisms responsible for illnesses and death in humans. Many of these pathogens cannot live and develop in an acid medium such as lactic acid. This powerful bactericidal property of fermented-milk products has been recognized by people in many parts of the world. Doubtless, lactic acid, as a bactericide, has played a vital role in maintaining health in the absence of sanitation and refrigeration.

In yogurt, *Salmonella typhi* die within thirty to forty-eight hours. *Escherichia coli* (*E. coli*) are unable to develop. *Salmonella paratyphi* and *Corynebacterium diptheriae* lose their pathogenic qualities. A long list of other virulent pathogens also are inhibited or killed after being introduced into cultured-milk products.

Yogurt has been found to have other benefits, too. It is useful in restoring the beneficial flora in the human intestinal tract that have been lost due to antibiotic treatment for an illness. Also, regular yogurt consumption helps to maintain health in the intestinal tract. Yogurt alleviates chronic constipation, and its use is preferable to repeated dosing with over-the-counter laxatives.

It is easy to make yogurt at home. Many cookbooks offer directions. Also, good-quality commercial yogurts have become available. Select full-fat, unflavored, organic yogurt. Read the label carefully for other important information. The cultures used to convert milk into yogurt are *Lactobacillus bulgaricus* and *L. thermophilus*. Also, some dairies add other cultures that are not needed for culturing but which add more benefits. Common ones include *L. acidophilus, L. bifidus, L. casei,* and *L. reuteri.*

Look for a statement on the label that the cultures are still active (or viable). A tricky phrase is "made with active cultures." Of course, the yogurt *must* be made with active cultures. But this does not necessarily mean that the cultures are still active. Some products are further heat treated to extend their shelf life. This practice destroys the cultures and is unnecessary. Yogurt has a relatively long shelf life. Look for the date on the label. Check the containers in the refrigerated cabinet. Frequently, stock of perishable food is rotated, with the older containers closer to the front. Fresher yogurt may be at the back, so compare dates.

At home, refrigerate the yogurt and plan to use it within a few weeks. Although yogurt remains safe, its bacterial strength gradually declines. Discard any yogurt that has developed mold.

Do not depend on frozen-yogurt products, such as yogurt ice cream, to provide the same benefits as plain, full-fat yogurt. Freezing results in a decline of the live organisms that make yogurt beneficial. Also, such products include undesirable additions, such as sugars, colorings, and flavorings. Instead, add plain, whole-milk yogurt to fresh fruits or frozen unsweetened berries.

Cheeses

Cheeses, as well, are quality protein foods. Select natural cheeses, such as cheddar, Swiss, and Camembert. Avoid processed cheeses, such as American cheese, as well as those that are even more highly processed: "process cheese food" and "process cheese food spread."

Purchase full-fat cheeses. Check the date on the label. Cheeses marked "aged for more than sixty days" indicates that if the cheese is made from raw milk, the aging period allows for the growth of beneficial microorganisms that inhibit the growth of any pathogenic bacteria that might be present. Raw-milk cheeses are available. Many of them are from Europe and are artisanal and regional.

The FDA is considering safety regulations to extend the aging period, or to pasteurize the cheese, or even to prohibit its production and importation. Are such draconian measures warranted? Not according to Catherine M. Donnelly, professor of nutrition and food sciences at the University of Vermont in Burlington. She is an expert on bacterial pathogens. Donnelly believes that the FDA's proposals are misguided. She reported that pasteurization actually makes cheese *more vulnerable to contamination* by destroying its natural bacterial barriers. The acidity, salt content, and currently used process of aging raw cheese for sixty days under refrigeration eliminate the possibility of pathogen survival. The FDA enforces these safeguards.

Donnelly charges that the proponents of revised legislation used flawed studies to support their case. They made inaccurate measurements of the cheeses' ability to combat pathogens by inoculating the cheeses with multiple types of bacteria at levels that never would occur under normal conditions. In addition, the proposed revisions would ruin the fine flavors and textures of cheeses.

Dairy Products Are Not for Everyone

Individuals who are truly allergic to milk need to avoid *all* dairy foods and *all* dairy components.

Individuals who have lactose intolerance (sometimes termed malabsorption)—a distinctly different problem from milk allergy—need to avoid or minimize dairy foods containing lactose, the milk sugar. In varying degree, such individuals lack lactase, the enzyme involved in metabolizing lactose. The condition ranges among individuals from a mild to a severe deficiency of lactase. After drinking dairy products containing lactose, the individual experiences discomfort, which may include abdominal pain, bloating, flatulence, and diarrhea.

Complete avoidance of dairy products may not be necessary for those with lactose intolerance. The more slowly that lactose-containing food is presented to the intestine, the more readily the lactose is digested and absorbed. Thus, consuming a small amount of milk along with solid food favors lactose absorption by delaying the gastric emptying of food from the stomach into the small intestine. Gastric emptying also is delayed in the presence of fats and amino acids. For these reasons, full-fat milk is tolerated better than skim milk. Also, nonfat milk solids may be added to skim milk to improve

HOW TO MAKE YOGURT CHEESE

Yogurt cheese is easy to make. It tastes like a good cream cheese.

Line a colander with cheesecloth and set the colander over a deep pot or a large bowl. Pour plain full-fat yogurt into the colander, cover with a clean dish towel, and allow the whey to drip overnight at room temperature. In the morning, carefully gather together the corners of the cheesecloth and tie them with a clean, strong cord. Remove the colander and suspend the hanging cheesecloth over the pot or bowl by means of a dowel, and allow additional whey to drip through. *Do not squeeze the cheesecloth.* After the whey stops dripping, carefully empty the contents of the cheesecloth into a container with a cover. This is cheese yogurt. Refrigerate and plan to use it within a few days.

You will find that a large amount of whey has separated from the curd (the cheese). You can drink it, add it to soups, stews, or vegetable juices, or refrigerate it in a tightly closed jar for future use. The whey will keep for several months. It makes an excellent starter for culturing vegetables. Or, if you cook whole-grain cereals, soak the grains overnight at room temperature in water and add some whey. The whey adds nutrients and improves the digestibility of the cereal.

its "skinny" texture. This addition increases the lactose content of the milk, making it more difficult for a lactose-intolerant individual to digest it. (A similar problem exists with low-fat cottage cheese. Nonfat milk solids may be added, which increases the level of lactose.)

Although fermented dairy products such as cheese, buttermilk, and yogurt have been recommended for lactose-intolerant individuals because the lactose is reduced in fermentation, not all of these foods are tolerated equally well. Some fermented cheeses, such as aged cheddar or Swiss, are significantly reduced in lactose because the whey, separated out from the curd, contains most of the lactose. On the other hand, the lactose level of other fermented dairy products, such as yogurt, cultured buttermilk, and sweet acidophilus milk, might be just as high as that of whole fluid milk. The lactose content of these products varies according to the processing technique.

Yogurt, with its bacterial beta-galactosidase (lactase) is tolerated better than regular fluid milk. Yogurt's bacteria survive gastric digestion and are active in the gastrointestinal tract. Hence, the bacteria can substitute for the individual's own lactase that might be low or lacking.

Cultured buttermilk does not change lactose digestion significantly because only a small amount of lactose is metabolized by its bacteria. For the same reason, the action of sweet acidophilus milk is equivalent to that of regular fluid milk; it does not alleviate the distressful symptoms for a lactose-intolerant individual.

Commercial food-grade lactases (beta-galactosidase enzyme preparations from microbial organisms) are used to produce lactose-hydrolyzed milk and other reduced-lactose products. They can be used instead of regular fluid milk. These products taste sweeter than regular fluid milk, but they contain from 40 to 90 percent less lactose. Such products are available from some dairies.

Another approach to making regular fluid milk better tolerated is to use lactose-reducing products. One is Lactaid, which is added to milk at home. To be fully effective, such products require a twenty-four-hour incubation period.

If you suspect that you are lactose intolerant, the condition can be confirmed at a hospital. Two diagnostic tests are available: One is an oral lactose-tolerance test, based on routine laboratory procedures. The other is a breath-hydrogen test, which is considered to be more reliable and useful in evaluating lactose digestion.

Apart from those who have milk allergy, lactose intolerance, or other conditions that may require milk avoidance, milk and cheese remain as good choices for quality protein.

Organ Meats

The British term organ meats "offal." Many Americans dub them "awful." There was a time, not long ago, when organ meats were plentiful in butcher shops. Regretfully, several factors have combined to make organ meats—except liver—virtually disappear from food stores.

There has always been some aversion to handling raw organ meats such as liver or kidney, due to their textures. In cooking kidneys, the strong unappealing odor can pervade the room. Liver has distasteful membranes. During the Depression years, organ meats, considered as byproducts, were affordable, while steaks, chops, and roasts were luxuries beyond lean budgets. Then, during the war years that followed, available meats were limited, but organ meats remained plentiful. Following World War II, steaks, chops, and roasts became available again, and were even affordable in the postwar boom. Organ-meat consumption, with its aversions and stigmas symbolizing lean economic times and war-sacrificing years, met another decline. At the same time, there was an increased interest in using these byproducts for pet foods and animal feeds. Although liver remained available, other organ meats became difficult to find in food stores.

Traditionally, dietitians had recommended that organ meats, especially liver, be eaten once a week. That advice was continued for many years. Then, the cholesterol scare burst on the scene. Wrongly, cholesterol-rich foods such as liver, eggs, butter, and cream were stigmatized as threats to heart health. In response, traditional dietitians revised their former recommendation. The new advice was that liver should not be eaten more than once a month and, if eaten, should be consumed in a very small amount!

This revision was unscientific. Cholesterol-rich foods do *not* raise blood cholesterol levels. If they are excluded from the diet, the body manufacturers even *more* cholesterol! It has taken years and overwhelming evidence to convince traditional health professionals, including dietitians, that cholesterol-rich foods, eaten regularly, are beneficial rather than harmful. Slowly, the maligned egg has been somewhat restored to its former positive and deserved image. Perhaps, in time, the formerly held high regard for liver will be restored, too. Both eggs and liver are among the most nutrient dense of all foods.

Because liver acts as a filter in the body, it excretes many toxins. However, excessive amounts of toxins may be stored in this organ. For this reason, it is important to find sources of wholesome livers from organically raised animals. Such sources are limited and difficult to find. If you cannot locate any, consider, as a second choice, selecting baby beef liver; the young animal has not lived long enough to accumulate high levels of toxins. Rotate liver consumption from calf to lamb or pork. Lamb is mild, while pork is strong flavored. Although chicken liver may be the tastiest, limit your consumption of chicken liver to those that are derived from organically produced birds. Conventionally raised chickens are fed arsenic compounds. Although there is a required time period for drug withdrawal before the chickens are marketed, arsenicals are found routinely in chicken livers when they are tested.

Some health conditions require the avoidance of liver. Individuals suffering from gout or other conditions that require a diet low in purines need to limit or avoid organ meats, as well as other foods rich in purines, such as muscle meats, seafood, lentils, peas, and beans.

Certain organ meats, especially brain, should not be eaten by anyone. At present, brain appears to be a risky organ involved with bovine spongiform encephalopathy (BSE), popularly termed "mad cow disease." Other high-risk organs and animal parts include the skull, trigeminal ganglia, eyes, vertebral column, spinal cord, and dorsal root ganglia of cattle aged thirty months or more, and the tonsils and small intestine of cattle of all ages. These constituents have been used in an industrial process known as "advanced meat recovery" (AMR) that removes muscle tissue from the bone of beef carcasses under high pressures, and the resulting product may be labeled as "meat." In December 2003, the USDA proposed to prohibit the use of brain, spinal cord, trigeminal ganglia, and dorsal root ganglia from cattle aged thirty months or more in "meat" produced by AMR, in order to minimize the risk of exposure to the BSE agent. Also, in order to reduce the risk of portions of the brain being dislocated into the tissues of the carcass as a result of stunning cattle before slaughter, the USDA's Food Safety and Inspection Service proposed a ban on air-injection stunning of animals.

For individuals on a rotation diet, it is possible to obtain liver from animals other than domesticated ones. Two companies in particular offer such a service, affording a greater diversity of liver from various animal species. For meats that can be shipped, contact Seattle's Finest Exotic Meats, 17532 Aurora Ave., North, Shoreline, WA 98133, (800) 680-4375, www.exotic meats.com; or Hills Foods Ltd., Unit 1-130 Glacier St., Coquitlam, BC, Canada V3K 5Z6; (604) 472-1500; www.hillsfoods.com. These groups supply organic meats, game meats, exotic meats, and specialty poultry.

As omnivores, we humans can choose highly nutritious organ meats. We can learn a lesson by observing the carnivores. When they kill, they eat the organ meats first.

Muscle Meats

The three main muscle meats popular with most Americans are beef, pork, and lamb. Other muscle meats, including goat, buffalo, and rabbit, are eaten to a far less extent. Depending on location, some people still hunt, kill, and eat antelope, bear, beaver, caribou, deer, elk, moose, muskrat, opossum, rabbit, raccoon, squirrel, and other wild animals.

Beef, pork, and lamb are consumed by most Americans so frequently that many Americans have developed allergies to these meats—especially beef and pork. Beef allergy is among the top ten allergens in America. For individuals who adhere to a diversified rotary diet, in order to lessen allergic reactions or to prevent them from developing, there are sources of alternative animal protein foods, offering meats from less utilized animal species such as bison, ostrich, reindeer, and wild boar. (See the section on organ meats for contact information.)

Beef, pork, and lamb are all quality protein foods, if tolerated. Through breeding programs, producers have been able to produce animals with significantly reduced fat in the carcasses to meet consumer preferences.

In selecting beef, pork, or lamb, look for meat with the USDA organic seal. If not available, second best is meat labeled "natural." This term signifies that the meat (or poultry) has met three USDA requirements: The product must contain no added coloring or artificial ingredients. The product must be only "minimally processed," as entailed in cutting, grinding, canning, drying, or freezing (traditional techniques to make food edible or to preserve it). The label must carry an explanation for the term "natural" after the name of the food, such as "no added coloring or artificial ingredients; minimally processed."

In addition, the USDA has approved other label claims, such as how animals were raised ("raised without hormones or antibiotics" or "fed grain grown without the use of pesticides"). All claims must be accurate and documented.

Free-range, grass-fed animals have less total fat than those fed grain. Also, the fat of free-range animals has more omega-3 fatty acids (low in the diet) and less omega-6 fatty acids (abundant in the diet). In composition, free-range animals approximate the wild animals consumed by hunter-gatherers. About two-thirds of the calories consumed by hunter-gatherers consisted of wild animals, and those people thrived, with low rates of heart disease.

Steaks, roasts, and chops are preferable to ground meats, unless the ground meats are from certified organic animals. Most bacteria spread more readily across the surface of meat instead of burrowing deep inside. When meat is ground its surface area is increased and spread across each long strand that comes out of the grinder. Any bacteria that were present on the original surface of the meat are mixed throughout the ground batch. Then, later, in forming patties, the original surface area is spread further, throughout the patties. In addition, ground meat may come from many different animals, even from animals raised in many different locations. If one animal is contaminated, the contamination can be spread through large volumes, and also be widely distributed. If organic ground meat is unavailable, select a whole piece of boneless meat and request the butcher to grind it to your order. Make certain that the grinding equipment is clean. Or, purchase a whole piece of boneless meat and grind it at home. Old-fashioned hand grinders are still available. (Contact The Vermont Country Store, P.O. Box 6999, Rutland, VT 05702; 802-362-8460; www.vermontcountrystore.com.) Or, use a food processor.

Handle all raw meat carefully. Follow the same safety practices with wrappings, cutting board, implements, and hand washing as previously described for poultry.

There are some myths regarding meats that need to be dispelled. Here are a few:

Myth 1: "Meat fats are unhealthy." All dietary fats, including meat fats, are healthy, provided they are not overconsumed, or heavily grilled so they char. Dietary fats, including those found in meats, play essential roles in the body. They are the most concentrated sources of food energy, providing more than twice as many calories per gram as do proteins or carbohydrates. Fats play roles in growth and in disease prevention.

Fats are vital as major components of all cell membranes, and they have important functions in biochemical regulation systems. They serve as precursors for beneficial compounds, such as prostaglandins, steroid hormones, and bile acids. Also, fats serve as thermal insulation for the body, protecting internal organs against shocks.

Fats are the major sources of vitamins A, D, E, and K (known as the fat-soluble vitamins), and fat consumption improves the absorption of these vitamins from foods. Fats also provide essential fatty acids such as alpha-linolenic and linoleic acids.

Myth 2: "Out with wooden cutting boards; in with plastic cutting boards." Not so fast. Ever since the introduction of plastic cutting boards it was assumed that they were impervious, could be cleaned thoroughly, and were more hygienic than porous wooden cutting boards. This untested assumption led the USDA, as well as many home-economics experts, to urge homemakers to choose plastic over wood, and for sanitarians to endorse plastic cutting boards for commercial settings.

In 1993, unexpected findings were reported in *Chemical & Engineering News* by microbiologists at the Food Research Institute of the University of Wisconsin at Madison. With concerns about the increasing problems of food-borne illnesses, Dean O. Cliver and Nese O. Ak attempted to find ways to decontaminate wooden cutting boards and make them as safe as plastic ones. To their surprise, they discovered that pathogens disappeared on wood, but thrived on plastic!

Cliver and Ak purposely contaminated 5-centimeter blocks from both plastic and wooden cutting boards with two nonpathogenic strains of *Escherichia coli*, the virulently pathogenic strain *E. coli 0157:H7*, *Listeria innocus*, *L. monocytogenes*, or *Salmonella typhimurium*. They reported that "bacteria inoculated onto plastic blocks were readily recovered for minutes to hours and would multiply if held overnight." However, "Recoveries from wooden blocks were generally less than those from plastic blocks, regardless of new or used status; differences increased with holding time." Clean wood blocks usually absorbed the inoculum completely within three to ten minutes. If the fluids contained the amount of bacteria likely to come from raw meat or poultry, the bacteria generally could not be recovered after entering the wood. At much higher levels, the bacteria might be recovered after twelve hours at room temperature and with high humidity, but their numbers were reduced by at least 98 percent and more often by more than 99.9 percent. The small remainder was removed readily with hot water and detergent. Cliver and Ak concluded that "cross contamination seems unlikely if the bacteria cannot be recovered by the procedures used in these experiments."

Surprised by their results, the researchers repeated the experiments several times. Each time, after exposure of only three minutes, in each type of wood tested, more than 99.9 percent of the bacteria disappeared. Yet, all bacteria on plastic surfaces survived. Old knife-scarred wood performed as well as new wood in its antibacterial effect. Yet, similarly scarred plastic seemed to encourage bacterial growth, which even survived scrubbing with soap and hot water!

In 1994, Cliver and Ak, joined by C. W. Kaspar, did additional studies with blocks of plastics, hard rubber, and nine different hardwoods. Bacteria were applied in a nutrient broth or chicken juice. They were then recovered by pressing the blocks onto agar as a nutrient. Bacteria inoculated onto plastic blocks were readily recovered after minutes to hours. They multiplied when held overnight. Recovery of bacteria from the wooden blocks generally was less than from the plastics.

Although new plastic-cutting-board surfaces were relatively easy to clean and were microbiologically clear, plastic boards with extensive knife scars were difficult to clean manually, especially if they had chicken fat deposits on them. Cleaning of the wooden boards with hot water and detergent generally removed remaining bacteria, regardless of bacterial species, wood species, and whether the wood was new or old.

Additional follow-up tests were performed by microbiologists at the University of Michigan. Viable bacteria were detected on wooden cutting boards when they were scanned with an electron microscope. But the researchers concluded that as long as surfaces were maintained in a hygienic fashion and sanitized frequently, there would be no danger of cross-contamination either from a wooden or a plastic cutting board.

In early 1997, Cliver, joined by P. K. Park, updated the findings of the University of Michigan tests. They, too, used an electron microscope and studied three types of plastic cutting boards. The scanning revealed new surprises. The plastic cutting boards had holes, grooves, punctures, and cavities that could shelter bacteria from manual cleaning. Polyethylene and foamed polypropylene were found to contain holes and perforations, even when the plastics were new. During normal use these surfaces acquired large numbers of deep knife-mark grooves, punctures, and cavities. Although acrylic cutting boards acquired fewer knife marks, with use they became much more splintered and fractured. All three surfaces were inoculated with a nutrient broth containing *L. monocytogenes, Staphylococcus aureus,* and *E. coli.* Vigorous washing with detergent and hot water failed to remove the bacteria from cavities in the boards. Dried bacteria deposits formed a biofilmlike attachment to the surface of the acrylic boards. These results help explain the findings that used plastic surfaces are more difficult to clean manually than old wooden surfaces.

The final word on cutting boards probably has not been made. Meanwhile, whatever type of cutting board you choose to use, keep it clean. Wash it with hot, soapy water, especially after it has been used for handling raw flesh foods. Allow the board to air-dry, or use clean paper towels. Sanitize it frequently by using a solution of 2 teaspoons of chlorine bleach in 1 quart of water. Rinse it well in clear water.

If possible, invest in two cutting boards. Reserve one for cutting raw flesh foods and the other for cutting all other foods, such as bread, raw vegetables, and raw fruits. By using separate cutting boards, you prevent cross-contamination. Play it safe.

Myth 3: "Pork—the other white meat." Is this slogan by the pork industry justified? No! The phrase exploits a widely held misconception that "red meat" such as beef or lamb is less healthy than "white meat" such as chicken or fish. The slogan is merely a gimmick intended to increase sales, and to present a more favorable image of pork.

What are the facts? The lack of redness in raw chicken and pork is attributable to a lack of a protein, myoglobin, which is present in all muscle meats, along with its relative, hemoglobin. Both myoglobin and hemoglobin bind oxygen. Myoglobin stores oxygen in cells; hemoglobin transports oxygen from the lungs to cells throughout the body.

On average, beef contains more myoglobin in its tissue than other types of meat. Beef contains 8 milligrams of myoglobin per gram (mg/g) of meat; lamb, 6 mg/g; pork, 2 mg/g; and poultry, 1–3 mg/g. The age of the animal affects its myoglobin content. Veal contains as little as 2 mg/g; and beef from old cattle, 18 mg/g. Processing, packaging, and cooking of the meat also affect its myoglobin content, which in turn affects its color. A fresh-cut pork chop is pinkish red; when vacuum-packed, purple; a cured pork chop, pink; and a cooked pork chop, white! Myoglobin levels also may vary within an animal, depending on muscle use. This feature accounts for light and dark meat in poultry. Because chickens do not fly, meat in their wings and breasts store little myoglobin. These sections are lighter in color than their legs and thighs, which are exercised more extensively. Also, the legs and thighs are closer to the bone, where there are more blood vessels.

Meat specialists advise consumers to purchase raw pork cuts that are pinkish red. Packaged pork that appears almost white tends to be dry and tough.

Myth 4: "Beef patties are safe to eat when, after being cooked, the red turns pink or brown." Color is a poor indication of beef's doneness and safety.

Raw ground beef oxidizes when exposed to air, causing the pink pigment to turn brown. This is apt to occur when raw ground beef has been stored in the refrigerator for some time, or when it has been frozen and then left to thaw for some time in the refrigerator. On the other hand, cooked ground beef may remain pink even when it has been cooked above 160°F. Even after beef has been cooked, it may retain pinkness due to the meat's pH (a measurement indicating relative acidity or alkalinity), the amount of pigment in the meat, or the beef's fat content.

For these reasons, the USDA now recommends the use of an instant-readout digital meat thermometer near the end of the cooking time for beef patties. Use this procedure: Check the indentation on the stem of the instrument to find out how deeply it needs to penetrate the patties for an accurate reading. Insert the thermometer into the thickest part of the patties. If the patties are not thick enough to check them from the top, insert the thermometer sideways. Remember that the safety point for cooked beef patties is 160°F.

Although use of the meat thermometer is recommended officially, consumers can still judge doneness in cooked beef patties by other observations. The cooked meat should be brown in the middle of the patties, and the cooked-out juice should be clear.

There is still another snag. The cooked color can be used as a safety indicator only if the patties are 100 percent beef. Sometimes ingredients such as starch, carrageenan, and soy protein are added to ground beef to reduce the fat percentage on the label. With such formulations, beef patties may turn brown before they reach a temperature sufficiently hot to ensure that all pathogenic bacteria are killed. Also, some butchers blend ground beef with ground pork or lamb. Exercise care to cook these mixed-meat patties thoroughly, especially if pork is included. Thorough cooking ensures that all live *Trichinella spiralis,* if present, are killed. This pathogenic organism is responsible for trichinosis. Again, play it safe!

If you have access to bones from organically raised animals, make good use of them. Place the bones in a pot, cover with water, add a small amount of vinegar to extract calcium from the bones, and simmer. Add this liquid to soup or stew. If the bones have marrow, extract and eat this valuable food. In former times, marrow was cherished. In the nineteenth century, a common practice was to add a marrow-extracting implement to a table setting. The marrow, spread on bread, was relished.

SEEKING QUALITY PROTEIN FOODS

Select fresh or frozen meats from well-raised animals. Avoid highly processed meat forms, such as frankfurters, luncheon meats, and meat products that have been pickled or brined (for example, corned beef), or those that have been cured, smoked, and nitrated (for example, ham).

Smoked protein foods, such as meats, fish, poultry, and cheeses, have become popular in restaurants, homes, and in marketed food products. Although many people enjoy the smoked flavor, the smoking process coats foods with polycyclic aromatic hydrocarbons (PAHs). These are carcinogenic compounds that are also found in cigarette smoke. Consumption of smoked foods, especially heavily smoked ones, are best avoided or limited.

LOWER-QUALITY PROTEIN FOODS

Beans, also known as legumes, are whole foods that can confer certain benefits, but they should not be regarded as good-quality protein foods. Beans have been a staple in the diet of many people, with the decline of hunting and gathering and the rise of agriculture. Beans grow readily and when dried can be stored for long periods of time.

Beans are good sources of dietary fibers. Also, they can help normalize blood sugar in persons with type 2 diabetes and blood fats in heart patients. However, when regarded as protein foods, beans have a lower quality than protein foods derived from animal sources. Beans either are low or lacking in one or more essential amino acids. To compensate for the deficiency or deficiencies, people may add small amounts of good-quality protein food to bean dishes. One example is the addition of ham to bean soup.

The Drawbacks of Beans

There are several drawbacks of beans. They are difficult to digest, and they produce flatulence. Humans lack an enzyme in the intestinal mucosa that is needed to split the oligosaccharides (long-chain sugars) present in beans. Instead, oligosaccharides remain in the intestinal tract where bacteria metabolize them and form large amounts of carbon dioxide, hydrogen gas, and small amounts of methane—all excreted in wind. This problem does not exist in foods derived from animal sources.

All raw legumes (beans and lentils) contain antinutrients, substances that can inhibit the proper absorption of nutrients. Raw peas, for example, contain lathyrogens, substances that can disrupt the structure of collagen in the body. Lathyrism, a disease in humans, is characterized by muscular weakness and paralysis in the lower part of the legs. Lathyrism has been recognized since the time of Hippocrates.

Many beans contain hemagglutinins, antinutrients that have the ability to agglutinate (clump together) the red blood cells in humans and other animals, and suppress growth significantly. Hemagglutinins combine with the cells that line the intestinal wall and interfere with intestinal absorption of nutrients.

The trypsin inhibitor is another antinutrient found in legumes. It prevents action of the enzyme trypsin, found in the digestive tract of humans and animals, from digesting and assimilating proteins properly. The trypsin inhibitor renders protein virtually worthless. *This condition persists, regardless of increased protein intake.* If these antinutrients are consumed constantly at high levels in the diet, they can lead to chronic health problems. In addition, trypsin normally allows vitamin B_{12} (cyanocobalamin) to be assimilated. Thus, by blocking trypsin activity, foods with the trypsin inhibitor increase the requirements for vitamin B_{12} and actually can create a deficiency of this vitamin. Levels of both hemagglutinin and the trypsin inhibitor are reduced somewhat by cooking legumes that contain these antinutrients. Protein foods from animal sources do not contain these antinutrients.

Two legumes deserve more detailed discussion, because both are in common usage and both present health problems. One is the peanut (a legume, not a true nut), and the other, the soybean.

Peanuts

Although the peanut is nutritious, this legume is overused. Allergic reactions to the peanut have increased in the United States by 95 percent over a recent ten-year period. This rise parallels the common practice of offering the seemingly benign peanut butter and jelly sandwich to very young children.

Unlike some food allergies, peanut allergy generally persists into the adult years. Peanut allergy is thought to be the leading cause of anaphylaxis, a violent allergic reaction that involves a number of parts of the body simultaneously, and can result in death. This serious and severe reaction occurs only after an individual has had previous experiences with the same allergen.

According to the FDA, as little as one-fifth to one-five-thousandth of a teaspoon of an offending food, such as peanut, has caused death from anaphylactic shock. Peanuts have been implicated in numerous cases of anaphylaxis, and many cases have been fatal.

Peanut allergy is one of the most severe of all food allergies. If a person becomes sensitized, there is no insignificant level of exposure. For example, a spatula used to remove peanut-containing cookies from a pan, and then used to remove peanut-free cookies from another pan, can render the latter cookies hazardous to a peanut-allergic individual. Similar cross-contamination can occur with shared ice-cream scoops, utensils, and machinery used both for products with and without peanuts.

Allergic reactions to peanuts can occur through skin contact, such as a kiss bestowed by someone who has eaten peanuts. The reaction can occur by inhalation. An airplane had to make an emergency landing because a peanut-allergic passenger reacted violently to the peanut dust released when other passengers opened peanut snack bags. Airlines have since switched from peanuts to pretzels as snack food. Some schools forbid children to bring peanut butter sandwiches in their bagged lunches because allergic children have reacted.

Soybeans

The soybean, like the peanut, is a legume. Among all of the legumes, it has the highest nutritional offerings. However, the soybean, like all beans, has a lower quality of protein than foods from animal sources. The soybean has been overrated and overused. As a result, it has become a major allergen. In addition, the soybean has many characteristics that make it far from being an ideal food.

The raw soybean, like other beans, contains numerous antinutrients. Although processing can reduce them, it does not eliminate them. The raw soybean is an anticoagulant (an agent that prevents blood clotting). This property is not reversed by vitamin K, which is a highly effective blood-clotting agent found in leafy green vegetables and liver. Many Americans are low in vitamin K. Soy's anticoagulant property is attributed to its antitrypsin activity.

The raw soybean contains other antinutrients, including phytic acid (also present in whole grains, as discussed in Chapter 3), which binds and prevents mineral absorption, especially zinc, calcium, and magnesium. Thus, vegetarians who consume high levels of soybeans and many soy-containing products, as well as phytate-containing grains, are at great risk of being deficient in these minerals. Phytates are present in plant foods but not in animal foods.

Hemagglutinins, discussed earlier, are present in the raw soybean. These antinutrients are reduced somewhat by cooking, but they still are present at lower levels. The only satisfactory method known at present to deactivate these antinutrients is traditional fermentation. This process involves a slow chemical change, triggered by bacteria, molds, and yeast. Fermentation deactivates the enzyme inhibitors, trypsin inhibitors, phytic acid, hemagglutinins, and vitamin antagonists present in raw soybeans. The fermentation process renders the nutrients present in soybeans more available and digestible. Unfortunately, the fermentation process is used with only a few soybean products, and they are not especially familiar nor readily available in American cuisine. The main fermented soybean products are tempeh (a soybean-based entrée), miso (a soybean paste used in soups and sauces), and natto (fermented whole soybeans). Tempeh and miso are available in many health/natural food stores in the United States. Natto, common in Japan, is unfamiliar and unavailable to most Americans. Natto is reported to have a strong odor, a sticky texture, and generally is not favored by novices. Because miso is used as a flavoring only, the sole fermented soybean food that is an acceptable dish is tempeh.

Contrary to popular notions, soybean products such as tofu and bean curd—familiar and available to Americans—are *not* fermented. Rather, they are processed by precipitation. This method deactivates *some* but *not all* of the antienzyme agents, and deactivates *only a little* of the phytates.

Soybeans, even processed ones, have antithyroid properties. The estrogenic isoflavones (particular plant pigments) in soy—genistein and daidzein—are much touted for their health benefits. What is unpublicized is that they are antithyroid agents. Individuals who consume soybean products habitually (the recommendation currently in vogue) may encounter long-range thyroid disturbances. Animal studies relate the isoflavones in soy to thyroid disorders, including goiter. Other studies relate soybean consumption not only to hypothyroidism, but also to low energy levels, poor mineral absorption, and infertility.

Even at exceedingly low levels, hormones can exert profound biological effects, either beneficial or detrimental. The estrogenic isoflavones in soy are being promoted enthusiastically as health promoters. Although they appear to *prevent* breast cancer if supplied early, they may *promote* breast cancer at a later stage. Both human and animal studies suggest that soy may *increase* the risk of breast cancer.

How beneficial are soy products being offered to Americans? The antinutrients in modern soy products, including soy flour, can inhibit animal growth. In humans, they can cause intestinal problems, reduce protein digestion, and lead to chronic deficiencies in the uptake of amino acids.

Textured soy protein, an inexpensive filler, became popular at one time as a hamburger extender. Presently, it is used extensively in processed foods, despite the fact that it contains antinutrients. On food labels, textured soy proteins may be designated as an ingredient by the acronym TSP.

Protein isolates from soy are used in powder mixes intended for meal-replacement drinks. These isolates are obtained by means of a high-temperature process that denatures the protein extensively. In its damaged form, the protein is rendered low in nutritional value. Soy protein (and other protein isolates) cause negative calcium balance in humans and other animals, and can contribute to the development of osteoporosis. Soy protein isolates are still high in mineral-blocking phytates, thyroid-depressing phytoestrogens, and potent enzyme inhibitors. Also, the high heat used in processing the isolates has been reported to increase the likelihood of carcinogenic compound formation.

Soy "milk" is used as a replacement for cow's milk and is marketed for the general population. Also, it is used as a substitute for cow's milk in infant-feeding formulas intended for babies who are allergic to cow's milk. Soy milk is *not* the equivalent of milk from humans (or from cows, goats, or sheep). Soy milk has several undesirable features when used in infant-feeding formulas. Soy can exert adverse effects on the hormonal development of infants. Soy-milk formula is devoid of cholesterol, a vital substance for proper development of the brain and central nervous system in infants. One study of infants given soy formula showed a concentration of estrogenic compounds as much as 22,000 times higher than those in infants fed breast milk or milk-based formulas. This startling finding caused speculation in the *New Zealand Medical Journal* that such an overload of estrogen in infants might result in precocious development of breast and secondary sex characteristics in very young females. In addition, it raised concerns that such an overload might result in male organs not developing normally at puberty.

Since the FDA approved a health claim for soy, more than a thousand new soy-containing products have flooded the marketplace, adding to the already existing plethora. Infants fed soy-milk formulas in order to avoid cow's milk allergy frequently develop allergy to soy. As soy is promoted aggressively and is available in increasing numbers of food and beverage products, the number of soy-allergic individuals is likely to increase due to a lifetime of soy overconsumption, unless one chooses basic foods and avoids processed ones. Even then, some soy may be in the diet, indirectly, from soy constituents in the feed of farm animals and farmed fish.

The soy health claim now permitted is based on 25 grams of soy protein daily, alleged to reduce the risk of heart disease. Such a daily overload of soy inevitably increases the risk of soy allergy and other problems. The FDA determined that diets with four daily servings of soy protein can reduce levels of LDL cholesterol. However, four daily servings of soy protein would promote the risk of more allergenic reactions, in addition to replacing high-quality protein foods that contain no antinutrients. Furthermore, the recommendations narrow the food base and negate the sound principle of choosing from as wide a variety of basic foods as possible.

The FDA's approval of the health claim was in response to a petition by a leading soy producer. The soybean lobby exerts powerful clout. The food and beverage processors favor greater soybean use because it is a low-cost filler, extender, and replacement in foods for humans and in feeds for animals. It is a cost cutter that swells profits. No other dietary staple has so many antinutrient drawbacks as soy. Conversely, no other food has so many public relation firms and lobbyists working for it.

Viewed sociologically, we have an ironic development regarding beans. Much of the world's population, especially in developing countries, struggles to include meat and other animal foods in diets that consist largely of beans. Animal foods are highly prized by such people, but they are too costly or not readily available for daily use. They are used infrequently, and only for special occasions. Such populations yearn to add animal foods to their diets.

On the other hand, people in developed industrialized countries—even those who are not affluent—have easy access to a wide variety of good-quality foods from animal sources. Yet, many individuals have chosen to limit or avoid these foods. Instead, they purposely follow diets that depend heavily on beans and grains. We can only conclude that people in the developing countries are following traditional dietary wisdom. Those in the developed countries have been misled by false official pronouncements, lobbyists, and advertising hype.

Moving Forward with a Whole Foods Diet

D o not become fanatical. As the eminent British physician Franklin Bicknell cautioned, "wholism" may be carried to an extreme. In *Chemicals in Food and in Farm Produce* (Faber &Faber, 1960), Bicknell facetiously describes wholism as "the philosophy of eating the whole of foods . . . [for example] the hooves, horns, and hide of the steer, with the sirloin." However, try to select whole foods that are basic. These are the ones that would have been familiar to our ancestors through the millennia. Whole foods have made it possible for humankind to survive, be healthy, and procreate. Only recently, and within a relatively brief span of time, have highly processed food forms been developed. They have low nutritional values, but high market profits. They are untrustworthy for the continuance of humankind's survival, health, and procreation.

Select as great a variety of foods as possible. Choose fresh, fully ripened produce, and eat it when it comes into its peak of flavor and nutrients. The wider the variety of foods you choose, the greater is the possibility you will obtain all essential nutrients and achieve a balance.

Food processing steers us in the opposite direction, limiting variety. For example, by using one food (wheat, corn, or soy) as a base, a manufacturer can create a dozen breakfast cereals that are all essentially the same, except for different shapes, colorings, flavorings, and product names. The "variety" offered by these products is illusionary. Similarly, fast-food restaurants, with their limited menus, curtail the range of offerings. Kale, broccoli, or artichokes are not apt to be on the menu. People who frequently eat at such places are narrowing their food base to the detriment of their health.

Quality whole foods are available. They will become more readily available as consumers become more enlightened about them and recognize their worth. Consumer interest assures producers of a receptive market and encourages them to raise quality foods. This trend leads to improved agricultural practices, with healthier crops and animals, and healthier people who consume them. Improved agricultural practices also result in less environmental degradation and pollution. Everyone wins: our land, animals, people, and our planet Earth.

Selected
References

Chapter 1

Adams, Catherine F. *Nutritive Value of American Food in Common Units*. Washington, D.C.: USDA Agricultural Research Service, Agricultural Handbook No. 456, Nov. 1975.

Agarwal, Sanjiv. "Tomato Lycopene and Its Role in Human Health and Chronic Disease." Reprinted from the *Canadian Medical Association Journal* in *Food Processing's Wellness Foods* (May 2001): 12–14.

Agarwal, Sanjiv, and A.V. Rao. "Tomato Lycopene and Low-Density Lipoprotein Oxidation: A Human Dietary Intervention Study." *Lipids* 33 (1998): 981–984.

Angier, Natalie. "Benefits of Broccoli Confirmed as Chemical Blocks Tumors." *New York Times* (Apr. 12, 1994): C11.

"Are All Veggies Created Equal?" *Food Product Design* (Nov. 2002): 20.

"Avocadoes Contain Potent Liver Protectants, Say Researchers." *Food & Chemical News* (Dec. 20, 2000): 6.

Associated Press. "New Evidence of Vegetables as Beneficial, Antioxidants Found to Combat Disease." *New York Times* (Nov. 9, 1994): A21.

Brody, Jane E. "A New Look at an Ancient Remedy: Celery. A Chemical in the Plant Lowers Blood Pressure in Animals." *New York Times* (June 9, 1992): C3.

———. "Eat Your Vegetables! But Choose Wisely." *New York Times,* (Jan. 2, 2001): D6.

Carroll, Martha Filipic. "Darker Vegetables Get an 'A'." Press release. Ohio State University, *Chow Line* (Apr. 2, 1998).

Coulombe, Roger. "New Wrinkles in the Plant-Cancer Connection." *Utah Science* 55; 3&4 (Fall/Winter, 1994): 12.

"Cruciferous Vegetables." Press release. University of New Hampshire, Cooperative Extension Service, undated.

Danzig, Laurie B. "The Whole Tomato? New Research on Breast Cancer Reveals the Importance of Synergy between Tomato Lycopene and Other Tomato Phytonutrients." *Food Processing's Wellness Foods* (Jan. 2002): 35–37.

Delaquis, P.J. and G. Mazza. "Antimicrobial Properties of Isothiocyanates in Food Preservation." *Food Technology* (Nov. 1995): 73–84.

Ennen, Steve. "Tomatoes Gain Strength in Cancer Battle." *Food Processing's Wellness Foods* (Nov/Dec. 2002): 18–21.

Fallon, Sally. "Fermented Vegetables and Fruits." In *Nourishing Traditions*. 2nd ed. Washington, D.C.: New Trends Publishing, 1999: 89–111.

Filipic, Martha. "Darker-leafed Lettuce Has More Vitamins." Press release. Ohio State University, *Chow Line* (Mar. 18, 1999).

———. "Seeing Red? That's Good If It's Lycopene." Press release. Ohio State University, *Chow Line* (Apr. 6, 2003).

Foltz-Gray, Dorothy. "Squash: As Good as Gold." *Health* (Jan./Feb. 1997): 30, 34–35.

Fortino, Denise. "A Boost for Broccoli." *Food & Wine* (June 1992): 118.

Fountain, Henry. "Pesticide Breakdown." Observatory column. *New York Times* (Sept. 28, 2004): F3.

"Garlic Prevents Plaque . . . But Lack of Standardized Extracts Foils Clinical Studies." *JAMA* 288; 11 (Sept. 18, 2002): 1342.

Gupta, N.P., and R. Kumar. "Lycopene Therapy in Idiopathic Male Infertility." *Food Processing* (July 2001): 40.

Hall, Trish. "Broccoli, Hated by a President, Is Capturing Popular Votes." *New York Times* (Mar. 25, 1992): C1, 6.

Hamlin, Suzanne. "The New Greens and How to Use Them." *New York Times* (Aug. 17, 1994): C1.

Harder, B. "Eat Broccoli, Beat Bacteria: Plant Compound Kills Microbe behind Ulcers and a Cancer." *Science News* (June 1, 2002): 340–341.

Haytowitz, David B., Ruth H. Matthews, et al. *Composition of Foods: Vegetables and Vegetable Products, Raw, Processed, Prepared*. Washington, D.C.: USDA Human Nutrition Information Service, Agricultural Handbook No. 8-11, revised Aug. 1984.

Huang, Mou-Tuan. "Super Phytochemicals." *The Energy Times* (Mar./Apr. 1995): 32–33.

Hunter, Beatrice Trum. *Favorite Natural Foods*. New York, NY: Simon & Schuster, 1974.

———. *The Natural Foods Primer: Help for the Bewildered Beginner*. New York, NY: Simon & Schuster, 1972.

Ingegno, Christianne. "Vintage Vinegar." *Food Product Design* (Oct. 2004): 144.

Kiple, Kenneth F., and Kriemhild Coneè Ornelas. *The Cambridge World History of Food*. 2 vols. New York, NY: Cambridge University Press, 2000.

Lipkin, Richard. "Vegemania: Scientists Tout the Health Benefits of Saponins." *Science News* 48 (Dec. 9, 1995): 392–393.

Pool-Zobel, B.L., et al. "Consumption of Vegetables Reduces Genetic Damage in Humans: First Results of a Human Intervention Trial with Carotenoid-rich Foods." *Carcinogenesis* 18 (1997): 1847–1850.

"Powerful Anticarcinogen Found in Onions." American Chemical Society, *What's Happening in Chemistry?* (1990): 37.

Raloff, Janet. "Studies Suggest How Salad May Protect Heart." *Science News* (June 23, 2001): 391.

————. "The Heart-Healthy Side of Lycopene." *Science News* (Nov. 29, 1997): 348.

Schildhouse, Jill. "The Almighty Garlic." *Food Product Design* (Mar. 2003): 14, 17.

Schloss, Andrew. "Broccoli Is Just the Beginning: The Rest Is a Family Affair." *Washington Post* (May 13, 1992): E1, 4.

Schneider, Elizabeth. "Broccoli & Co." *Food Arts* (Sept. 1996): 75–81.

————. "Chicory & Co." *Food Arts* (Mar. 1993): 68–71.

————. "Squash Games." *Food Arts* part 1 (Oct. 2000): 205–212; part 2 (Oct. 2001): 168–175.

————. "Tender Squashes of Summer." *Food Arts* (Apr. 2001): 192–201.

"Study Says Tomato May Limit Cancers." *New York Times* (Apr. 13, 1999): D8.

Tannahill, Reay. *Food in History.* New York, NY: Stein & Day, 1973.

Terry, M.P.H., et al. "Brassica Vegetables and Breast Cancer Risk. Letters. *Journal of the American Medical Association* 285; 23 (June 20, 2001): 2975–2976.

Uhl, Susheela. "It's Easy Being Greens." *Food Product Design* (May 2003): 144.

————. "The Cucurbits—Pumpkin, Squash and Gourd." *Food Product Design* (May 2001): 156.

————. "Vegetables Underground." *Food Product Design* (Nov. 2001): 122.

"Vegetables and Fruits Found to Curb Stroke in Men." *New York Times* (Apr. 12, 1995): A1.

Wang, L. "Veggies Prevent Cancer through Key Protein." *Science News* (Mar. 24, 2001): 182.

Chapter 2

Adams, Catherine F. *Nutritive Value of American Food in Common Units.* Washington, D.C.: USDA Agricultural Research Service, Agricultural Handbook No. 456, Nov. 1975.

Almada, Anthony. "Pomegranates and Vascular Health." *Functional Foods and Nutraceuticals* (Nov. 2004): 66.

Altman, Lawrence K. "Not Just for Refreshment Anymore: Grapefruit Juice Is a Topic of Study." *New York Times* (Feb. 19, 1991): C3.

"Apples Help Prevent Cancer." *Food Product Design* (Aug. 2001): 18.

"Berry Anthocyanins Are Effective Antioxidants." *Food Product Design* (Nov. 1999): 143.

"Berry, Berry Good for You." *Food Product Design* (Nov. 2000): 144.

"Berry Extracts May Inhibit Cancer." *Food Technology* (Feb. 2002): 10.

"A Blue Nutraceutical." *Prepared Food's Nutra Solutions* (Sept. 2001): NS19.

"Blueberries Rated as Having Highest Antioxidant Capacity." *Food Technology* (June 1999): 158.

"Breathe Easier with Apples." *Food Product Design* (Mar. 2002): 27.

Broihier, R.D., Kitty, "Get the Most from the Blues." *Food Processing* (July 2000): 53–54.

"Bye-Bye 'Prunes.' Hello 'Dried Plums.'" *Food Product Design* (Oct. 2000): 19.

Carroll, Martha Filipic. "Antioxidants Fight Free Radicals." Press release. Ohio State University, *Chow Line* (Aug. 20, 2004).

———. "Apples Are Healthy to the Core." Press release. Ohio State University, *Chow Line* (May 15, 1997).

———. "A Banana a Day: A Good, Healthy Snack." Press release. Ohio State University, *Chow Line* (May 15, 1997).

———. "Cranberries Not a Typical Garden Crop." Press release. Ohio State University, *Chow Line* (Nov. 26, 2000).

———. "Forget the Suds, Use Water to Wash Fruit." Press release. Ohio State University, *Chow Line* (May 28, 1998).

———. "Fruit Lasts Longer in the Refrigerator." Press release. Ohio State University, *Chow Line* (Oct. 22, 1998).

———. "Research Could Be Berry Good News." Press release. Ohio State University, *Chow Line* (June 10, 2001).

———. "Watermelon: Plenty of Reasons to Enjoy." Press release. Ohio State University, *Chow Line* (Aug. 8, 1996).

"Cherries." *Prepared Foods* (Nov. 2002): 60.

"Cherries Chock Full of Benefits." *Food Product Design* (Jan. 1998): 31.

"Chokeberry Combines Nutrition with Return to Tradition." *Food Product Design* (July 1997): 108.

"Dried Plums Kill Bacteria." *Food Product Design* (Nov. 2001): 21.

Farnsworth, N.R., et al. "Potential Value of Plants as Sources of New Antifertility Agents." *J Pharm Sci* 64 (1975): 717–754.

Foster, R.J. "Fruit's Plentiful Phytochemicals." *Food Product Design* (Sept. 2004): 75–81.

Frank, Paula. "Research Reveals Additional Health Benefits of Apples." *Stagnito's New Products Magazine* (June 2001): 21–26.

Gebhardt, Susan E., Rena Cutrufelli, Ruth H. Matthews, et al. *Composition of Foods: Fruits and Fruit Juices, Raw, Processed, Prepared*. Washington, D.C.: USDA Human Nutrition Information Service, Agricultural Handbook No. 8-9, revised Aug. 1982.

"Grape Compound with Anticancer Activity." *Chemical & Engineering News* (Jan. 13, 1977): 20.

Gray, Paula. "Figs." *Hanover (N.H.) Coop News* (Feb. 2003): 12.

Hamilton-Miller, J.M.T. "Reduction of Bacteriuria and Pyuria Using Cranberry Juice." Letters. *JAMA* 272 (Aug. 24–31, 1994): 8; followed by letters on same topic by Roger Goodfriend, M.D., Walter J. Hopkins, Ph.D., et al., Louis M. Katz, M.D., Jerry Avorn, M.D., et al., and Michael J. Haverkorn, M.D., Ph.D.: 588–590.

"Infection Fighters in Cranberries Identified." *Chemical & Engineering News* (Oct. 2, 2000): 45.

Jang, Meishieng, Lining Cai, George O. Udeani, et al. "Cancer Chemopreventive Activity of Resveratrol: A Natural Product Derived from Grapes." *Science* 275 (Jan. 10, 1997): 218–220.

Joseph, James A., and Barbara Shukitt-Hale. "Blueberry Elixir Reverses Age-Related

Symptoms." USDA Agricultural Research Service, *Agricultural Research* 48; 2 (Feb. 2000): 23.

"Juicy Anticancer Prospects." *Science News* 149 (May 4, 1996): 287.

Kilham, Chris. "Health Benefits Boost Elderberry." *Prepared Foods* (June 2001): 39.

Kiple, Kenneth F., and Kriemhild Coneè Ornelas. *The Cambridge World History of Food*. 2 vols. New York, NY: Cambridge University Press, 2000.

Kolettis, Helen. "The Goodness of Grapes." *Food Product Design* (Sept. 2003): 14, 16.

LaBell, Fran. "Antioxidants Isolated from Tart Cherries." *Prepared Foods* (June 1998): 97–98.

———. "Raisins—Sweetness, Functionality and Nutrition." *Prepared Foods* (Nov. 2000): 91.

"Link Found between Cranberry Juice and Heart Health." *Food Technology* (May 2003): 10.

Maas, John L. "Strawberry Varieties Rich in Ellagic Acid." USDA Agricultural Research Service, *Food & Nutrition Research Briefs* (Oct. 1997): 1.

Magee, James B. "Muscadine Grapes: New Health Food?" USDA Agricultural Research Service, *Food & Nutrition Research Briefs* (Jan. 1998): 1.

McCandless, Linda. "Antioxidant Activity of Apples Is High." Cornell University's College of Agriculture and Life Sciences, *Cornell Focus* 8; 2 (Aug. 1999): 3.

"Orange a Day Keeps Cancer Away." *Food Product Design* (Jan. 2004): 29.

Prior, Ronald L. "Blueberries Not Equal in Antioxidant Power." USDA Agricultural Research Service, *Food & Nutrition Research Briefs* (Jan. 1999): 3.

———. "Spinach 'n Strawberries—An Antioxidant Recipe." USDA Agricultural Research Service, *Food & Nutrition Research Briefs* (July 1997): 2.

Raloff, Janet. "Berry Promising Anticancer Prospects." *Science News* (May 6, 2000): 298.

———. "Watermelon: Red Means Lycopene Rich." *Science News* (July 13, 2002): 29.

"Raspberry-Rich Diet Forestalls Cancer in Rats. *Science News* 151 (Apr. 11, 1998): 239.

Rimando, Agnes. "Therapeutic Berries?" USDA Agricultural Research Service, *Agricultural Research* 49; 9 (Sept. 2001): 23.

Schildhouse, Jill. "Bravo for the Avocado." *Food Product Design* (Food Service Annual) (Apr. 2003): 52.

Seppa, Nathan. "Researchers Find How Rhubarb Remedy Eases Cholera." *Science News* (Mar. 30, 2002): 205.

Streiff, Richard. "Folate Levels in Citrus and Other Juices." *American Journal of Clinical Nutrition* 24; 2 (Dec. 1971): 1390–1392.

"Study a Boon for Prunes." *Food Product Design* (May 1999): 20.

"Superfood of the New Millennium." Hillsborough County Newsletter, University of N.H. Cooperative Extension Service (July/Aug. 2000): 1, 3.

"Take Two Tart Cherry Pills..." *Food Product Design* (Mar. 1999): 20.

Tannahill, Reay. *Food in History*. New York, NY: Stein & Day, 1973.

Tucker, Katherine. "Fruits and Vegetables Build Strong Bones, Too." USDA Agricultural Research Service, *Food & Nutrition Research Briefs (July 1999): 1–2.*

Uhl, Susheela. "Berry Berry Good." Food Product Design *(Jan. 2002): 110.*

Wedge, David E. "Berries Curb Cancer Cells." *USDA Agricultural Research Service,* Agricultural Research *50; 6 (June 2002): 23.*

Chapter 3

Ashby, John K. "The Grain, the Whole Grain, and Nothing But . . . " *Food Processing's Wellness Foods* (Jan./Feb. 2004): 30–34.

Behall, Kay. "Grains Lay Claim to Health Gains." USDA Agricultural Research Service, *Agricultural Research* (May 2003): 8–9.

Bliss, Rosalie M. "A Grain of Truth about Fiber Intake." *Agricultural Research* (Dec. 2004): 16.

Brody, Jane E. "For Unrefined Healthfulness: Whole Grains." *New York Times* (Mar. 4, 2003): F5, 8.

Chatenoud, Liliane C., La Vecchia, S. Franceschi, et al. "Refined-Cereal Intake and Risk of Selected Cancers in Italy." *American Journal of Clinical Nutrition* 70 (1999): 1107–1110.

Drake, Dennis L., Susan E. Gebhardt, Ruth H. Matthews, et al. *Composition of Foods: Cereal Grains and Pasta, Raw, Processed, Prepared.* Washington, D.C.: USDA Human Nutrition Information Service, Agricultural Handbook No. 8-20, revised Oct. 1989.

"Eat Your Oatmeal." *Stagnito's New Products Magazine* (May 2002): 66.

Filipic, Martha. "Whole Grains a Whole Lot Better." Press release. Ohio State University, *Chow Line* (July 14, 2002).

Fung, T.T., F.B. Hu, M.A. Pereira, et al. "Whole Grain Intake and the Risk of Type 2 Diabetes: A Prospective Study in Men." *American Journal of Clinical Nutrition* 76 (Sept. 2002): 535–540.

Gordon, Dennis. "Whole-Grain Health Claim Needs Improvement." *Food Technology* (June 2003): 244.

"A Grain of Truth About Fiber Intake." USDA Agricultural Research Service, *Agricultural Research* (Dec. 2004): 16.

Gråsten S.M., K.S. Juntunen, K.S. Poultanen, et al. "Rye Bread Improves Bowel Function and Decreases the Concentration of Some Compounds That Are Putative Colon Cancer Risk Markers in Middle-Aged Women and Men. *Journal of Nutrition* 130 (Sept. 2000): 2215–2221.

Harden, Ben. "Wholesome Grains, Insulin Effects May Explain Healthful Diet. *Science News* (May 18, 2002): 308–309.

Hazen, Cindy. "Food for Better Health." *Culinology* (Nov. 2004): 22, 25.

Hirsch, Julie B., and Yanni Papanikoloau. "Getting a Lignan—(or Is It Lignin?)—Up on Health." *Food Processing's Wellness Foods* (July/Aug. 2002): 31–33.

Hunter, Beatrice Trum. *The Family Whole-Grain Baking Book.* New Canaan, CT: Keats Publishing, 1973.

———. *Gluten Intolerance.* New Canaan, CT: Keats Publishing, 1987.

————. *Grain Power.* New Canaan, CT: Keats Publishing, 1994.

————. *Wheat, Millet and Other Grains.* New Canaan, CT: Keats Publishing, 1982.

————. *Whole-Grain Baking Sampler.* New Canaan, CT: Keats Publishing, 1972.

Jacobs, David, et al. "Is Whole Grain Intake Associated with Reduced Total and Cause-Specific Death Rates in Older Women?" *American Journal of Public Health* 89 (Mar. 1999): 107–109.

Kagnoff, Martin, K.A. Raleigh, J.J. Hubert, et al. "Possible Role for a Human Adenovirus in the Pathogenesis of Celiac Disease." *Journal of Experimental Medicine* 160 (Nov. 1984): 1544–1557.

Kiple, Kenneth F., and Kriemhild Coneè Ornelas. *The Cambridge World History of Food.* 2 vols. New York, NY: Cambridge University Press, 2000.

Liu, Simin, J.E. Manson, M.J. Stampfer, et al. "A Prospective Study of Whole-Grain Intake and Risk of Type 2 Diabetes Mellitus in U.S. Women." *American Journal of Public Health* 909 (Sept. 2000): 1409–1415.

————. "Whole Grain Consumption and Risk of Ischemic Stroke in Women: A Prospective Study." *Journal of the American Medical Association* 284; 12 (Sept. 27, 2000): 1534–1540.

McKeown, N.M., J.B. Meigs, et al. "Whole-Grain Consumption." *American Journal of Clinical Nutrition* 76 (Aug. 2002): 390–398.

"More Good News for Grains." *Food Product Design* (Apr. 1999): 32.

"Oatmeal Linked to Better Memory." *Food Product Design* (Jan. 2002): 22.

Orlando, Michael. "Whole Grains Go Mainstream." Guest editorial. *Food Product Design* (Oct. 2004): 17, 19.

Pereira, Mark A., et al. "Effects of Whole Grains on Insulin Sensitivity in Overweight Hyperinsulinemic Adults." *American Journal of Clinical Nutrition* 75 (May 2002): 848–855.

Pins, J.J., et al. "Do Whole-Grain Oat Cereals Reduce the Need for Antihypertensive Medications and Improve Blood Pressure Control?" *Journal of Family Practice* 51 (2002): 353–359.

Slavin, Joanne L., David Jacobs, Len Marquart, et al. "The Role of Whole Grains in Disease Prevention." *Journal of the American Dietetic Association* 101; 7 (July 2001): 780–785.

Slavin, Joanne L., and David Kritchevsky. "Pass the Whole-Grain Snack Food, Please." *Food Technology* 56; 5 (May 2002): 216.

Spiller, Gene and Monica. *What's with Fiber?* Laguna Beach, CA: Basic Health Publications, 2005.

Tannahill, Reay. *Food in History.* New York, NY: Stein & Day, 1973.

"A Tasty Source of Whole-Grain Nutrition." *Food Product Design* (Feb. 2003): 108.

Toops, Diane. "Whole Grains Can Cut Insulin and Cholesterol." *Food Processing's Wellness Foods* (Nov./Dec. 2002): 12.

Wade, Marcia A. "White Bread? Whole Grain Instead?" *Prepared Foods* (Nov. 2004): 53.

"Whole Grains Lower Heart Disease Factors." *Food Processing's Wellness Foods* (July/Aug. 2002): 13.

"Whole Grain Lowers Both Ischemic Stroke and Type 2 Diabetes." Egg Nutrition Center, *Nutrition Close-Up* 17; 4 (winter 2000): 4.

"Whole Grains to Go Mainstream." *Food Product Design* (Dec. 2003): 24.

"Wholesome Whole Grains." *American Institute for Cancer Research Newsletter* 78 (winter 2003): 4.

Chapter 4

Abbey, M., et al. "Partial Replacement of Saturated Fatty Acids with Almonds or Walnuts Lowers Total Plasma Cholesterol and Low-Density Lipoprotein Cholesterol." *American Journal of Clinical Nutrition* 59 (May 1994): 995–999.

Aber, R., et al. "Dermatitis Associated with Cashew Nut Consumption—Pennsylvania." Center for Disease Control & Prevention, *Morbidity and Mortality Weekly Report* 32; 9 (Mar. 11, 1983): 129–130.

Adams, Catherine F. *Nutritive Value of American Food in Common Units.* Washington, D.C.: USDA Agricultural Research Service, Agricultural Handbook No. 456, Nov. 1975.

Alday, E., et al. "Occupational Hypersensitivity to Sesame Seeds." *Allergy* 51; 1 (Jan. 1996): 69–70.

"Almonds Add Nutritional and Sensory Value." *Food Product Design* (Oct. 2000): 139.

"Almonds Might Inhibit Cancer." *Food Product Design* (July 1999): 26.

Associated Press. "Study Concludes that Eating Nuts Can Cut the Risk of Heart Attack." *New York Times* (Mar. 4, 1993): B8.

Bower, B. "Almond Joy, Stone-Age Styles: Our Ancestors Had a Bash Eating Wild Nuts." *Science News* (Feb. 23, 2002): 117.

Brewer, Helen Dean. "Today's Tree-Nut Craze." *Food Product Design* (May 2003): 14, 19.

Burrington, Kimberlee J. "Simply Nuts." *Food Product Design* (Mar. 2001): 101–117.

Burros, Marian. "Where Indulgence Grows on Trees." *New York Times* (Jan. 13, 1999): D1, 4.

"Cashew Oil May Conquer Cavities." *Science News* (Mar. 23,1991): 191.

Choate, R.D., Mary S. "Nutty about Nuts." *Hanover* (N.H.) *Co-op News* (Nov. 2000): 6.

Dahm, Lori. "Nuts Make a Comeback: The Latest Nutrition Research Propels Nuts to the Forefront of Good-for-You Foods." *Stagnito's New Products Magazines* (Sept. 2002): 38–39.

"FDA Approves Qualified Health Claim for Nuts." *Food Product Design* (Aug. 2003): 24.

Fernández, C., et al. "Allergy to Pistachio: Cross-Reactivity Between Pistachio Nut and Other Anacardiaceae." *Clinical & Experimental Allergy* 25; 12 (Dec. 1995): 1254–1259.

Filipic, Martha. "Be on Watch for Nutty Health Claims." Press release. Ohio State University, *Chow Line* (Sept. 7, 2003).

———. "Not All Pine Nuts Are the Same." Press release. Ohio State University, *Chow Line* (Sept. 2, 2001).

———. "Nothing Nutty about This Idea." Press release. Ohio State University, *Chow Line* (Jan. 27, 2002).

————. "Throw Out Cashews? Some People Do." Press release. Ohio State University, *Chow Line* (Dec. 8, 2002).

"Focusing on the 'Nut' in Nutrition." *Food Product Design* (July 1998): 31.

Gallo-Torres, Julia M. "The Almighty Almond." *Prepared Foods* (July 2002): 44.

Hamlin, Suzanne. "Walnuts: Good Taste, Good Fat." *New York Times* (Sept. 28, 1994): C1, 6.

"Health Benefits of Almonds." *Food Product Design* (July 2002): 29.

"Highlighting Hazelnuts." *Food Product Design* (Dec. 1998): 109.

Frazer, G.E., et al. "A Possible Protective Effect of Nut Consumption on Risk of Coronary Heart Disease: The Adventist Health Study." *Arch Intern Med* 152 (1992): 1416–1424.

Hirsch, Julie B. "Crazy for Nuts." *Food Processing* (Mar. 2003): 44.

Hirschwehr, Reinhold, et al. "Identification of Common Allergenic Structures in Hazel Pollen and Hazelnuts: A Possible Explanation for Sensitivity to Hazelnuts in Patients Allergic to Tree Pollen." *Journal of Allergy & Clinical Immunology* 90; 6 (Dec. 1992): 927–936.

Hu, F.B., et al. "Frequent Nut Consumption and Risk of Coronary Heart Disease in Women: Prospective Cohort Study." *British Medical Journal* 317 (1998): 1341–1345.

Jansen, M.D., et al. "Allergy to Pistachio Nuts." *Allergy Proceedings* 13; 5 (Sept./Oct. 1992): 255–258.

Jaret, Peter. "Good News in a Nutshell: Feel a Snack Attack Coming On? Go Ahead and Eat All the Nuts You Want." *Health* (July/Aug. 1996): 34, 36.

Jiang, Rui, JoAnn E. Manson, Meir J. Stampfer, et al. "Nut and Peanut Butter Consumption and Risk of Type 2 Diabetes in Women." *Journal of the American Medical Association* 288; 20 (Nov. 27, 2002): 2554–2560.

Juttelstad, Ann. "Nuts and Seeds Add Special Extras to Bakery Goods." *Baking Management* (Nov. 2001): 33–34, 36.

Kanny, G., C. De Hauteclocque, and D.A. Moneret-Vautrin. "Sesame Seed and Sesame Seed Oil Contain Masked Allergens of Growing Importance." *Allergy* 51; 12 (Dec. 1996): 952–957.

Kiple, Kenneth F., and Kriemhild Coneè Ornelas. *The Cambridge World History of Food.* 2 vols. New York, NY: Cambridge University Press, 2000.

Knight, Timothy E., and Björn M. Hausen. "Dermatitis in a Nutshell: Occupational Exposure to *Macadamia integrifolia.*" *Journal of the American Academy of Dermatology* 35; 3 (September 1996): 482–484.

Kolettis, Helen. "Nutty Nutrition—Almond Health Benefits." *Food Product Design* (Sept. 2003): 108.

LaBell, Fran. "Almonds Add Delicate Gourmet Touch." *Prepared Foods* (June 2003): 77.

————. "Consumers Crave Pistachios." *Prepared Foods* (Nov. 1996): 65.

————. "Nuts About Nutrition." *Prepared Foods* (Mar. 2001): 69–70.

Lavanish, J.M. "Biocidal Activity of Anacardic Acid from Cashew Fruit." Letters. *Chemical & Engineering News* (Dec. 17, 1984): 4.

Mann, George V. "Walnuts and Serum Lipids." Correspondence. *New England Journal of Medicine* 329; 5 (July 29, 1993): 358.

McCarthy, Marie A., Ruth H. Matthews, et al. *Composition of Foods: Nut and Seed Products, Raw, Processed, Prepared.* Washington, D.C.: USDA Human Nutrition Information Service, Agricultural Handbook No. 8-12, revised Sept. 1984.

Miraglio, Angela M. "Going Nuts about Nutrition." *Food Product Design* (Jan. 2003): 30, 33–34.

"New Studies Support Almond Nutrition." *Food Product Design* (June 2003): 30.

Noble, Holcomb B. "A Handful of Nuts and a Healthier Heart." *New York Times* (Nov. 17, 1998): D10.

Nordlee, Julie A., et al. "Identification of a Brazil-Nut Allergen in Transgenic Soybeans." *New England Journal of Medicine* 334; 11 (Mar. 14, 1996): 688–692.

"Nutty Way to Head Off Heart Disease." *Science News* (Mar. 13, 1993): 175.

Ohr, Linda M. "The Skinny on Beneficial Fats." *Prepared Foods* (Nov. 1998): 67–70.

"Pecans Rich in Vitamin E." *Food Product Design* (Oct. 2002): 29.

Perkins, Maggie Spirito. "Sesame Allergy Is Also a Problem." *British Medical Journal* 313; 7052 (Aug. 3, 1996): 300.

Pruess, Joanna. "Going to Seeds, Crunch, Crackle and a Hull Lot of Flavor." *Washington Post* (Jan. 19, 1994): E1, 4.

Pszozola, Donald E. "Health and Functionality in a Nutshell." *Food Technology* (Feb. 2000): 54–59.

Raloff, Janet. "Heart Risks: This Is Nutty." *Science News* (July 25, 1992): 52.

———. "High-Fat and Healthful, Scientists Offer a Nutty Recipe for Hale Hearts and Slim Physiques." *Science News* (Nov. 21, 1998): 328–330.

Rector, Sylvia. "Nutty Diets." *Journal Star* (Peoria, IL) (Dec. 5. 2001): C1–2.

Roux, N., S. Hogendijk, and C. Hauser. "Severe Anaphylaxis to Pine Nuts." *Allergy* 53; 2 (Feb. 1998): 213–214.

Sabaté, Joan, et al. "Effects of Walnuts on Serum Lipid Levels and Blood Pressure in Normal Men." *New England Journal of Medicine* 328; 9 (Mar. 4, 1993): 603–607.

Schneider, Elizabeth. "Chestnuts Revisited." *Food Arts* (Nov. 1993): 90–96.

———. "Pine Nuts, Beyond Pesto." *Food Arts* (Oct. 1995): 87–91.

"Sensational Sesame Seed." *Food Product Design* (July 2001): 27–28.

Sloan, A. Elizabeth. "About to Go Nuts." *Food Technology* (Feb. 1997): 18.

"Sunflower Kernels Replace Nuts with a Healthy Image." *Food Formulating* (Apr. 1995): 28–29.

Tannahill, Reay. *Food in History.* New York, NY: Stein & Day, 1973.

Toops, Diane. "Almond's Joy, Twenty Almonds a Day Keeps the Cardiologist Away." *Food Processing* (Oct. 2002): 59.

———. "In a Nutshell, Exotic Hazelnuts Combine Indulgence with Good Health." *Food Processing* (May 2003): 54, 56.

USDA Yearbook of Agriculture. *Seeds.* Washington, D.C.: U.S. Government Printing Office, 1961.

Yager, Brian. "Cooking Up Some Nutty Ideas." *Food Product Design* (Aug. 2003): 76, 78, 82, 85–86, 89.

Chapter 5

Adams, Catherine F. *Nutritive Value of American Food in Common Units.* Washington, D.C.: USDA Agricultural Research Service, Agricultural Handbook No. 456, Nov. 1975.

Anderson, Barbara A., Jeanne L. Lauderdale, I. Margaret Hoke, et al. *Composition of Foods: Beef Products, Raw, Processed, Prepared.* Washington, D.C.: USDA Human Nutrition Information Service, Agricultural Handbook No. 8-13, revised Aug. 1986.

Anderson, Barbara A., Marjorie L. Clements, Lynn E. Dickey, et al. *Composition of Foods: Lamb, Veal, and Game Products, Raw, Processed, Prepared.* Washington, D.C.: USDA Human Nutrition Information Service, Agricultural Handbook No. 8-17, revised Apr. 1989.

Constantinou, A. "Interaction Between Genistein and Estrogen Receptors May Enhance Mammary Tumor Growth." *American Association for Cancer Research* (Apr. 2000). Reported by L. Guterman in "The Power of Soy," *Today's Chemist at Work* (June 2000): 47.

Dees, C., et al. "Dietary Estrogens Stimulate Human Breast Cells to Enter the Cell Cycle." *Environmental Health Perspectives* 105 suppl 3 (1997): 84–85.

Divi, R.L., et al. "Anti-thyroid Isoflavones from Soybean." *Biochemical Pharmacology* 54 (Nov. 15, 1997): 1087–1096.

Exler, Jacob, et al. *Composition of Foods: Finfish and Shellfish Products, Raw, Processed, Prepared.* Washington, D.C.: USDA Human Nutrition Information Service, Agricultural Handbook No. 8-15, revised Sept. 1987.

Fisher, Marjorie. *Enjoy Nutritious Variety.* Winnetka, IL: Nutrition for Optimal Health Association, 1980.

Fort, P., et al. "Breast and Soy-Formula Feeding in Early Infants and the Prevalence of Autoimmune Thyroid Disease in Children." *Journal of the American College of Nutrition* 9 (Sept. 1990): 164–167.

Gaullier, J.M., J. Halse, K. Hoye, et al. "Conjugated Linoleic Acid (CLA) Supplementation for One Year Reduces Body Fat Mass in Healthy, Overweight Humans." *American Journal of Clinical Nutrition* 79 (2004): 1118–1125.

Haytowitz, David B., Ruth H. Matthews, et al. *Composition of Foods: Legumes and Legume Products, Raw, Processed, Prepared.* Washington, D.C.: USDA Human Nutrition Information Service, Agricultural Handbook No. 8-16, revised Dec. 1986.

Hesser, Amanda. "A Cutting Board with the Right Stuff." *New York Times* (Aug. 4, 1999): D3.

Hilakivi-Clarke, L., et al. "Maternal Exposure to Genistein During Pregnancy Increases Carcinogenic-Induced Mammary Tumorigenisis in Female Rat Offspring." *Oncology Report* 6 (Sept./Oct. 1999): 1089–1095.

———. "Maternal Genistein Exposure Mimics the Effects of Estrogen in Mammary Gland Development in Female Mouse Offspring." *Oncology Report* 5; 3 (May/June 1998): 609–616.

Hourihane, J. O'B., et al. "Clinical Characteristics of Peanut Allergy." *Clinical and Experimental Allergy* 27; 6 (June 1997): 634–639.

Hunter, Beatrice Trum. "Beneficial Bacteria." *Consumers' Research Magazine* (Jan. 1996): 8–9.

———. "Cutting Boards: Wood or Plastic?" *Consumers' Research Magazine* (Mar. 1998): 8–9.

———. "How Probiotics Fight Food-Borne Illness." *Consumers' Research Magazine* (Dec. 1993): 19–21.

———. "For Safe Palatable Meat—Use a Thermometer." *Consumers' Research Magazine* (Nov. 1997): 8–9.

———. "Lactose Intolerance." *Consumers' Research Magazine* (Mar. 1986): 8–9.

———. "Making Good Foods Better: Refashioning Eggs." *Consumers' Research Magazine* (July 2000): 26–31.

———. "Miss Muffet's Whey." *Consumers' Research Magazine* (Feb. 2003): 8–9.

———. "A Nutrient Low in the Modern Diet: CLA." *Consumers' Research Magazine* (Nov. 1998): 8–9.

———. "The Risk of Peanuts: Food Allergies, No Trivial Health Matter." *Consumers' Research Magazine* (Feb. 1999): 21–25.

———. *Yogurt, Kefir, and Other Milk Cultures.* New Canaan, CT: Keats Publishing, 1973.

Ikeda, T., et al. "Dramatic Synergism between Excess Soybean Intake and Iodine Deficiency on the Development of Rat Thyroid Hyperplasia." *Carcinogenesis* 4 (Apr. 21, 2000): 707–713.

Irvine, C., et al. "The Potential Adverse Effect of Soybean Phytoestrogens in Infant Feeding." *New Zealand Medical Journal* 108 (May 24, 1995): 318.

James, V. " Comments on Isoflavones in Soy-Based Infant Formulas." *Journal of Agricultural Food Chemistry* 46 (1998): 3395; also Comments, M.G. Fitzpatrick, 3396–3397.

Kiple, Kenneth F., and Kriemhild Coneè Ornelas. *The Cambridge World History of Food.* 2 vols. New York, NY: Cambridge University Press, 2000.

Lepkovsky, S. "Antivitamins in Foods." *Toxicants Occurring Naturally in Foods.* Washington, D.C.: National Academy of Sciences/National Research Council, pub. 1354 (1966): 98–104.

Liener, I.E. "Hemagglutinins in Foods." In *Toxicants Occurring Naturally in Foods* (pub. 1354). Washington, D.C.: National Academy of Sciences/National Research Council, 1966: 51–57.

Matone, G., et al. "Effects of Genistein on Growth and Development of the Male Mouse." *Journal of Nutrition* 86 (1956): 235–240.

McGuineness, J., et al. "The Effects of Long-Term Feeding of Soya Flour on the Rat Pancreas." *Scandinavian Journal of Gastroenterology* 15 (1980): 497–502.

Murphy, P.A. "Phytoestrogen Content of Processed Soybean Foods." *Food Technology* 36 (1982): 50–54.

Orum, B. "Nutritional Quality of Soybean Protein Isolates: Studies in Children of Preschool Age." In *Soy Protein and Human Nutrition.* New York, NY: Academic Press, 1979.

Petrakis, N.L., et al. "Stimulatory Influence of Soy Protein Isolate on Breast Secretion in Pre- and Post-Menopausal Women." *Cancer Epidemiology and Biological Previews* 5 (1996): 785–794.

Posati, Linda P., and Martha Louise Orr, et al. *Composition of Foods: Dairy & Egg Products, Raw, Processed, Prepared.* Washington, D.C.: USDA Human Nutrition Information Service, Agricultural Handbook No. 8-1, revised Nov. 1976.

Posati, Linda P., et al. *Composition of Foods: Poultry Products, Raw, Processed, Prepared.* Washington, D.C.: USDA Human Nutrition Information Service. Agricultural Handbook No. 8-5, revised Aug. 1979.

Rackis, J.J. "Biological and Physiological Factors in Soybeans." *Journal of the American Oil Chemists' Society* 51 (Jan. 1974): 161A–170A.

Raloff, Janet. "Wood Wins, Plastic Trashed for Cutting Meat." *Science News* (Feb. 6, 1993): 84–85.

———. "Family Allergies? Keep Nuts Away from Baby." *Science News* (May 4, 1996): 279.

Reese, K.M. "Remarks on Cutting Boards . . . " Newscripts. *Chemical & Engineering News* (Apr. 26, 1993): 88.

———. "Wooden Cutting Boards Safer Than Plastic Ones." Newscripts. *Chemical & Engineering News* (Mar. 1, 1993): 136.

Schroeder, Henry A. *The Poisons Around Us.* Bloomington, IN: Indiana University Press, 1974.

Setchell, K.D.R., et al. "Exposure of Infants to Phyto-oestrogens from Soy-Based Infant Formula." *Lancet* 350 (1997): 23–27.

———. "Isoflavone Content of Infant Formulas and the Metabolic Fate of These Phyto-estrogens in Early Life." *American Journal of Clinical Nutrition* 68, suppl. (1998): 1353S–1461S.

———. "Phytoestrogens: The Biochemistry, Physiology, and Implications for Human Health of Soy Isoflavones." *American Journal of Clinical Nutrition* 68, suppl. (1998): 1333S–1346S.

"Styrene Monomer Found to Migrate to Eggs During Storage." *Food Chemical News* (Apr. 29, 1991): 61.

Tannahill, Reay. *Food in History.* New York, NY: Stein & Day, 1973.

Wang, Y.M., et al. "Conjugated Linoleic Acid and Obesity Control: Efficiency and Mechanism." *International Journal of Obesity* 28 (2004): 941–955.

Zacharisen, Michael C., and Viswanath Kurup. "Anaphylaxis to Beans." *Journal of Allergy and Clinical Immunology* (part 1) 101; 4 (Apr. 1998): 556–557.

Index

Abbey, Mavis, 100
Acidophilus bulgaricus, 1
Acrylamide and starchy
    foods, 85–88
Adrenal hormones, 127
Advanced meat recovery,
    150
AgCanada, 42
Agricultural Research
    Center, Finland, 134
Ak, Nese O., 152–153
Alanine, 124
Albert, Christine, 97
Allergies. *See* Food
    allergies.
Almonds, 1, 95, 98–99,
    101–102, 103–104
Alpha-linolenic acid,
    97–98, 100–101, 114
American Association for
    World Health, 133
American Association of
    Cereal Chemists, 78
American Chemical
    Society, 45
American College of
    Cardiology, 60
American Dietetic
    Association, 110
American Heart
    Association, 72, 101
American Humane
    Society, 135
*American Journal of Clinical
    Nutrition*, 73, 133

*American Journal of Public
    Health*, 75
American Medical
    Association, Council,
    137
Amino acids, 119–127, 156
    functions of essential,
    120–123
    functions of
    nonessential, 123–127
Anaphylaxis, 158
Anthocyanins, 38, 39, 53
Anthocyanosides, 38
Anti-inflammatories, 52
Antimicrobial activity, 47
Antinutrients, 157–158
Antioxidants, 5, 38, 51,
    52–53, 62
    top-scoring vegetables
    for, 6
Antithyroids, 159
Apples, 1, 49–51
    juice, 50
Aretaeus, 89
Arginine, 94, 124
Armbruster, Gertrude, 30
Arnold, Dieter, 86
Artemis International, 39
Artichokes
    globe (French), 16–17
    Jerusalem, 17
Ascorbic acid. *See* Vitamin
    C.
Asparagine, 87
Aspartic acid, 124–125

Asthma, 49
Avocado, 12–14

Bacteria, 1, 33, 46, 47, 63,
    119, 135, 141–144,
    146–147, 151–155, 157
Bailey, David, 56
Bananas, 51–52
Barley, 1, 128
Baskin-Robbins, 47
Bean curd, 159
Beans, 16, 128, 156–161
    drawbacks of, 157
Beef, 53, 128, 150–156
    allergies, 150
    hamburgers, 53–55
    steak, 1
Beets, 6
    greens, 21
Bell peppers, red, 6
Berries, 5, 39–43
    distinguishing, 43
Beta-carotene, 13, 23, 24,
    25, 30, 38, 39, 45, 48, 51
Bicknell, Franklin, 163
Bilberries, 44, 46
Bioflavonoids, 38
Biological values of food,
    127–128
Blackberries, 41, 43
Blood pressure,
    high, 72
    whole grains and, 72
Blueberries, 41, 43, 44–46
Body mass index, 74

Bone growth, 121
Bovine spongiform
    encephalopathy (BSE),
    149
Boysenberry, 43
Brain metabolism,
    125–126, 140
Brain consumption,
    149–150
Braly, James, 91
Brand-Miller, Jennie, 84
Brazil nuts, 104
Breads, whole-grain, 80
Brigham and Women's
    Hospital, Boston, 102
    Division of Preventive
    Medicine, 73
Broccoli, 5, 6, 8
Brussels sprouts, 6
Bubel, Mike, 33
Bubel, Nancy, 33

Cabbage, 1, 5, 8, 34–36
    chinese, 21
    green or white, 21
    red, 21
    savoy, 21
Cadmium, 69
Calcium, 18, 68
Caldwell Bio-Fermentation
    Canada, 36
Calgene, 14
California Prune Board, 64
Calories, 95
Cancer, 4–5, 15, 20, 40,
    48–50, 55–56, 71
    colorectal, 71
    esophageal, 41
    nuts and, 101–102
    prostate, 101
    stomach, 71
Carbohydrates, 3, 70, 74,
    95, 131
Cardiovascular disease
    and nuts, 96–101
Cardoon, 18

Carnitine, 121
Carnosol, 5
Carotenoids, 5, 24, 38
Carroll, Kenneth K., 55
Carrots, 1, 8, 29
Cashews, 95, 105
Castaneda, Carmen, 130
Cauliflower, 8
Celeriac, 18
Celery, 1, 21
Celiac disease, 89
Cereals, whole-grain, 81–82
Champlain, Samuel de, 17
Chard, 7
Charlemagne, Emperor,
    113
Cheese, 145–146
    camembert, 145
    cheddar, 1, 145
    Swiss, 145
*Chemical & Engineering
    News*, 152
Chemical additives, 1
*Chemical in Food and in
    Farm Produce*, 163
Cherries, 41, 52–54
Cherry Marketing
    Institute, 52
Chestnuts, 105
Chia seeds, 133
Chicken, 1, 138–139
    feed studies, 133–134
    free-range, 134
    myths about, 139
    yellow vs white, 139
    See also Poultry.
Chicory, 21
Children, 51, 75–76, 124
Children's Hospital,
    Boston, 74
Chioffi, Nancy, 33
Chlorogenic acid, 38
Chlorophyl, 23
Chokeberry, 43
Cholesterol, 72, 97, 132,
    138, 149

high-density (HDL), 72,
    98, 100, 131–132
low-density (LDL), 39,
    55–56, 60, 72, 74, 98,
    100, 131–132, 161
very low-density
    lipoprotein (VLDL),
    132
Chromium, 68
Cigarette smoke, 125
Citrulline, 125
Citrus fruits, 5, 54–58
CLA, 143–144
Clemson University, 40
Clevidence, Beverly A., 61
Cliver, Dean O., 152–153
Coates, Gary, 54
Cobalamin. *See* Vitamin
    B$_{12}$.
Cobalt, 68
Coconuts, 106–107
Collagen, 124, 126
Commonwealth Scientific
    and Industrial
    Research
    Organization,
    Australia, 100
ConAgra Food
    Ingredients, 76
Conjugated linoleic acid.
    See CLA.
Conley, Susan Templin,
    139
Cook, Captain, 36
Cooking, 28–30
Copper, 68
Corn, 2, 6, 30, 128
Corn flakes, 2
Cornell University, 11, 30,
    51, 59, 93
    Department of
    Nutritional Sciences,
    30
    New York State College
    of Agriculture and
    Life Sciences, 59

Cortés, Hernandez, 14
Crackers, whole-grain, 81
Cranberries, 43, 46–47
Creasy, Leroy L., 59
Creatine, 126
Creighton University, NE, 61
Crim, Marilyn C., 130
Cucumber, 5
Cultured dairy products, 144–145
Curcumin, 5
Cutting boards, 152–154
Cysteine, 125
Cystine, 125

Dairy products, 51, 128, 142–148
   allergies to, 146–148
   fermented, 147
   reduced fat, 143
Dandelion leaves, 22
Dangerous Grains, 91
Davis, Paul A., 99–101
Deep Root Organic, 36
Detoxification, 5, 122
Dhiman, Tilak, 143
Diabetes, 17, 70, 73, 83
   whole grains and, 73
Diabetes, type 2, 73
Dichter, Ernest, 63
Dietary Guidelines for Americans, 2, 72
Donnelly, Catherine M., 146

E. coli, 45–47, 50, 64, 152, 154
Edwards, Alison J., 61
EFAs, 24–25
Egg Beaters, 137
Eggplant, 5, 6
Eggs, 1, 128, 132–138
   allergies to, 138
   alternative additive studies, 133–134

brown vs white, 135–136
   cartons, 134
   limiting consumption of, 136
   myths about, 135–138
   organic, 134–135
   substitues, 136–137
   whites vs yokes, 136
Eitenmiller, Ron, 108
Elderberry, 43
Ellagic acid, 38
Endive, Belgian or French, 22
Enig, Mary, 36
Environmental Protection Agency. *See* U.S. Environmental Protection Agency.
Enzymes, 88–89
   digestive, 88–89
Epicatechin, 38
Epithelial cells, 89
Escarole, 22
Essential fatty acids. *See* EFAs.
Estrogen, 5, 160
Exercise, 129

Fallon, Sally, 36
Fats, 3, 94–95, 109, 115, 152
   monounsaturated, 13, 94, 99, 103, 108, 118
   polyunsaturated, 94–95, 118
   saturated, 94–95, 106
   unsaturated, 94
Federal Institute of Health Protection of Consumers and Veterinary Medicine, Germany, 86
Fennel, 18, 22
Fermenting, 33, 159
Fiber, 48, 50, 67, 70, 84, 95, 109, 156

Filberts, 107
Fish, 128, 140–142
   depletion of wild, 140–141
   farming, 140–141
   oils, 134
   purchasing, 142
   raw, 142
   wild vs farmed, 141
Flatulence, 157
Flavr Savr, 14–15
Flavonoids, 5, 11, 38, 49, 61, 63
Flaxseeds, 1, 113–115
   ancient uses, 113
   oil, 24, 25, 113–114, 133–134
Florida Department of Citrus, 54
Flour, white, 2, 67–69, 77
   enrichment, 69, 77
Folate. *See* Folic acid.
Folic acid, 48, 55, 69
Folts, John, 60
Foo, L. Yeap, 46
Food
   bioengineered, 112
   intolerances. *See* Food allergies.
   measuring protein quality in, 127–129
   partitioning of, 2
   protein, 119–161
   smoked, 156
   See also Whole foods.
Food allergies, 20, 111–112, 138, 136, 150, 157–158
Food and Agricultural Organization (FAO), 88, 128
Food Guide Pyramid, 37–38, 77, 94 , 128–129
Food Product Design, 102
Food Processing's Wellness Foods, 78

Food Standards Agency,
Britain, 87
Framingham Heart Study,
74
Fraser, Gary E., 96
Free radicals, 5–6, 38–39,
125
Fruits, 2, 4, 14, 37–66
buying and storing,
65–66
citrus, 54–58
dried, 63–64
juices, 2, 37–38
top-scoring for
antioxidants, 41
See also individual types.
Fung, Daniel, 64

Gandhi, Mahatma, 113
*Garden Way's Guide to Food
Drying,* 33
Garlic, 10–11
General Mills, 76, 79
Georgetown University
Medical Center, 60
Gesher Benot Ya'aqov
(site), 93
Glucose, 87, 126
Glucose Revolution, The, 84
Glucosinolates, 5
Glutamic acid, 125
Glutamine, 126
Gluten sensitivity, 88–91
Glycemic index and whole
grains, 83–85
Glycine, 126
Glycogen, 123, 124
Goiters, 29
Goitrogens, 29
Gooseberries, 43
Gordon, Dennis T., 78
Goren-Inbar, Naama, 93
Grains, refined, 67–69
Grains, whole. *See* Whole
grains.
Grapefruit, 54

juice, 54, 56–57
pink, 41
Grapes, 58–61
juice, 59
muscadine, 58
red, 41
seeds, 61
Greene, Janet, 33
Growth hormone. *See*
Human growth
hormone.

Harvard University, 72, 75
Medical School, 97
School of Public Health,
96, 102
Hazelnuts, 107
Health and nuts, 95–103
Health Research and
Studies Center, Los
Angeles, 98
Health Professionals
Follow-Up Study, 73
Healthy People 2010, 72
Heart disease
protein and, 131
whole grains and, 71–72
Hebrew University, 93
Hemagglutinins, 157, 159
Hertzberg, Ruth, 33
Hesperidin, 38
High-density lipoprotein
(HDL). *See*
Cholesterol.
Hippocrates, 113
Histamine, 120
Histidine, 120
Hobson, Phyllis, 33
Food Guide Pyramid,
37–38, 77, 94
Hoggan, Ron, 91
Hollings Cancer Center,
SC, 48
Homocysteine, 131
Howell, Wanda, 133
Hu, Frank B., 96

Human growth hormone,
123, 126
Human Nutrition
Research Center on
Aging, 75

Immune system, 125
Indigestion, 90
Indoles, 5
Industrial Research, New
Zealand, 46
Infections, 20
Insulin, 74
resistance, 74–75, 83
International Chemical
Congress of the Pacific
Basin Societies 2000,
13
Inulin, 17, 63
Iron, 13, 18, 23, 68–69
Isoflavones, 38
Isoleucine, 121
Iowa Women's Health
Study, 98

Jacobs, David R., 75
Jacques, Paul, 74
Jang, Yangsoo, 71
Jansen, M.C.J.F., 71
Japan Ministry of
Education, 13
Jeffrey, Elizabeth, 5
Jenkins, David J.A., 80,
83–84
Joseph, James A., 45
*Journal of Agriculture and
Food Chemistry,* 6, 11
Journal of Food Science, 108
Journal of Nutrition, 136
*Journal of the American
Dietetic Association,* 67
*Journal of the National
Cancer Institute,* 101
Journal Star, Peoria, 93

Kagome, 13

Kale, 6, 7
Kanarek, Robin, 76
Kansas State University, 136
    Dept. of Animal Sciences and Industry, 64
Kasper, C.W., 153
Katelaer, Vincent, 89
Kawagishi, Hirokazu, 13
Kefir, 144–145
Keeton, Jimmy T., 64
Keeping the Harvest, 33
Kelp, 134
Kessler, David, 76
Khader, Dina, 80
Kidneys, 148
King's College, London, 49
Kiwi fruit, 41
Klebsiella, 20
Kohlrabi, 18–19
Krakanut, 110
Kris-Etherton, Penny, 101
Kresty, Laura Ann, 40, 48
Kummerow, F.A., 137

Lachance, Paul A., 37
Lactaid, 148
Lactases, 148
Lactic acid, 144
Lactobacillus fermentum, 46
Lactose intolerance, 146
Lamb, 150–156
    roast, 1
Lauric acid, 107
Learning and whole grains, 75
Lee, Chang Y., 49
Lee, Hyoung, 54
Leeks, 12
Legumes. *See* Beans.
Lettuce, 22–23
    bibb, 23
    Boston, 23
    iceberg, 23
    leaf, 23

romaine, 23
Leucine, 121
Lichtenstein, Alice, 96
Lima beans, 16
Limes, Tahiti, 55
Lind, James, 35
Linoleic acid, 25, 114
Lipids, 97, 131–132
Listeria innocus, 152
Listeria monocytogenes, 46, 64, 152, 154
Liu, Rui Hai, 11, 30, 51
Liu, Simin, 73
Liver, 1, 122, 128, 148–150
Loma Linda University, 96, 103
    School of Public Health, Dept. of Nutrition, 97
Loganberry, 43
Longevity and whole grains, 75
Louisiana Agricultural Experiment Station, 134
Low-density lipoprotein (LDL). *See* Cholesterol.
Lungs, 49
Lutein, 38
Lycopene, 15, 30, 38, 61–62
Lysine, 94, 120, 121

Macadam, John, 107
Macadamias, 95, 107–108
Magnesium, 52, 61, 68
Maillard reaction, 87
Malathion, 6
Manganese, 68
Marine environmental degradation, 141
Marrow, 156
Mattes, Richard, 103
Mayo Clinic, MN, 49
McKeown, Nicola, 75
McManus, Kathy, 102
Mead, Gretchen, 33
Meat, 148–156

free-range, 151
    muscle, 150–156
    myths about, 152
    organ, 148–150
    organic, 151
    raw, 151
Meat thermometers, 155
Medici, Catherine de, 16
Mediterranean diet, 97–98
Melons, 61–62
Mercury, 141
Methionine, 122, 131
Michigan State University
    Agriculture Experiment Station, 52
    Dept. of Horticulture, Bioactive Natural Products section, 52
    Natural Food Safety and Toxicology Center, 52
Midwest Advanced Food Manufacturing Alliance, 52
Milk products. *See* Dairy products.
Mills, Jan, 39
Milner, John, 101
Minerals, trace, 3
Mississippi State University, 58
Molybdenum, 68
Morgan, Wanda, 100
Mottram, Donald S., 87
Mueller, Ferdinand von, 107
Muscle meats, 150–156
Muscles, 121, 126
Mushrooms, shiitake, 134
Mustard, 5

Nair, Muralee, 52
National Academy of Sciences, Food and Nutrition Review Board, 95

National Broiler Council, 139

National Cancer Institute, 4, 29, 37

National Food Administration, Sweden, 86

National Institute on Aging, 45

National Institutes of Health, 97, 104, 133

National Research Council, 129

Native Americans, 115, 117

Natto, 159

Navidi, M.K., 137

Naylor, Rosamond L., 141

Nervous system, 121, 124, 127

Nestlé Research Center, Switzerland, 87

New England Journal of Medicine, 98, 104

New Zealand Medical Journal, 160

New Mexico State University, Las Cruces, 100

New York State Agricultural Station, Dept. of Food Services and Technology, 49

Niacin. *See* Vitamin B₃.

Nitrogen, 121

North Dakota State University, 78

Nottingham University, 49

Nourishing Traditions, 36

Nurses' Health Study, 72–73, 75, 96–97, 130–131

Nutrients and nuts, 94–95

Nutrition and Cancer, 71

Nuts, 93–112
allergies to, 111–112

buying and storing, 110–111
cancer and, 101–102
cardiovascular disease and, 96–101
cautions, 111–112
health and, 95–103
nutrients in, 94–95
obesity and, 102–103
types of, 103–110
See also individual types.

Oatmeal, 75–76, 81

Oats, 128

Obesity
nuts and, 102–103
whole grains and, 73–75

Offal. *See* Organ meats.

Ohio State University, 15
College of Medicine, 40, 48–49
James Cancer Hospital and Solove Research Institute, 40
Laboratory of Cancer Chemoprevention and Etiology, 40

Oils, 24–26
flaxseed, 24, 25
olive, 24–26
sesame seed, 116

Okamoto, Yasuko, 5

Okra, 19

Oldways Preservation Trust, 78

Omega-3 fatty acids, 24, 25, 95, 114, 133–134, 140–141

Omega-6 fatty acids, 24, 25, 114

Onions, 6, 11–12

ORAC test, 44

Oranges, 1, 41, 54
juice, 54, 56

Organ meats, 148–150

Ornithine, 126

Oxalic acid, 19, 28–29

Park, P.K., 153

Parsley, 23

Patulin, 50

Peanuts, 128, 157–158

Peas, 128

Pecans, 1, 95, 100, 108

Pennsylvania State University, 101

Peppers, 16

Pereira, Mark A., 74

Pesticides, 6

Phenolic compounds, 5, 42, 46

Phenols, 38

Phenylalanine, 122

Phenylketonuria, 122

Phloretin glycosides, 38

Phosphatides, 114

Phosphorus, 68

Physicians' Health Study, 97

Phytochemicals, 3–6, 38–39, 49, 55, 69–70

Phytonadione. *See* Vitamin K.

Piche, L.A., 131

Pickling, 33

Pignolia. *See* Pine nuts.

Pine nuts, 109

Pistachios, 1, 95, 109

Plaque, 47

Plums, 41
dried, 64

Pollution, Profits, and Progress, 67

Polyphenolic catechins, 5

Polyphenols, 38

Pomegranates, 62–63

Pork, 150–156
chops, 1, 155
muths, 154–155

Porta, Sepp, 42–43

Potassium, 13, 18, 51, 51, 61, 68, 106

Potatoes, 1–2, 8–9, 128
  chips, 2
Poultry, 138–140
  free-range, 138
  myths about, 139–140
  organic, 138
  See also Chickens.
Prebiotics, 63
Prepared Foods, 133
Preservatives, 1
Prior, Ronald L., 44
Proanthocyanadins, 38
Proanthocyanins, 45
Probiotics, 63, 144
Processed foods, 2
Produce for Better Health
  Foundation, 43
Proline, 126
Prostaglandins, 114
Protein, 3 , 94–95, 119–161
  animal sources vs plant
    sources, 128–129
  lower-quality food for,
    156–161
  measuring quality in
    foods, 127–129
  RDA for, 129–132
  re-examining
    requirements for,
    129–132
  selecting quality food
    for, 132–156
Protein efficiency ration
  (PER), 127–128
Protein digestibility-
  corrected amino acid
  scoring (PDCAAS),
  128
Protein isolates, 160
Prunes, 41, 63
Pseudomonas aeruginosa, 20
Pumpkin, 9–10
  seed, 1, 115
Purdue University, 103
Purines, 149
Purslane, 133

Putting Food By, 33
Pyridoxine. *See* Vitamin
  B$_6$.

Quercetin, 38, 48, 49–50
Quicksilver. *See* Mercury.

Radiation damage, 125
Radium, 104
Raisins, 41, 63
Rao, Venket, 15
Rappini, 10
Raspberries, 41, 43, 48–49
RDA. *See* Recommended
  dietary allowances.
Reaven, Gerald, 83
Recommended dietary
  allowances (RDAs),
  129
Rector, Sylvia, 93
Refining process, 1
Resveratrol, 38, 42, 58–59,
  60
Riboflavin. *See* Vitamin B$_2$.
Rice, brown, 1, 128
Root cellaring, 33
Root Cellaring, 33
Rosemary, 5
Royal Children's Hospital,
  Australia, 117
Rutin, 38
Rutgers University, 42, 45
Rye, 128
  berry, 1

Sabaté, Joan, 97
Sacks, Frank, 102
Salad dressing, 24–28
Salad greens, 20–23
  field, 22
  shopping for, 20–21
Salads, 20–21, 23–24,
  24–28
  non-greens in, 23–24
Salem, Norman, 133
Salmonella enteritidis, 135

Salmonella typhimurium,
  64, 152
Saponins, 15
Sauerkraut, 34–35
Schlundt, Jorgen, 86
Schroeder, Henry A., 67,
  143
Seeds, 93–94, 112–118
Selenium, 70, 104
Serine, 126
Serotonin, 123
Sesame seeds, 1, 115–117
  allergies to, 116–117
  oil, 116
Seventh-Day Adventists,
  96
Shallots, 12
Shellfish, 142
Shibamoto, Takayuki, 6
Shiitake mushrooms, 134
Shizuoka University, 13
Simon, Joel, 100–101
Simopoulos, Artemis P.,
  133
Slavin, Joanne L., 67, 75,
  78
Small Fruit Research
  Laboratory, MS, 58
Smoking. *See* Cigarette
  smoke.
Society for Neuroscience,
  76
Sodium, 68
Solar Food Dryer, 33
Soy, 158–161
  milk, 160
Soybeans, 112, 158–161
Sphera Foundation, 98
Spiller, Gene A., 98, 103
Spinach, 6, 7
Squalene, 25
Squash, 5, 9–10
  seeds, 115
Stabilizers, 1
Stadler, Richard H., 87
Stanford University,

Center for
Environmental Science
and Policy, 141
Medical School, 83
Staphylococcus aureus, 64,
154
Starches, 83, 85–88
Steaming, 30
Stir-frying, 30
Stockholm University, 75
Stoner, Gary, 40
Strawberries, 1, 41, 43
Streiff, Richard R., 55
Strokes
nuts and, 100–101
whole grains and, 72–73
Sugar, 46–47, 63
Sulfur, 5
Sunflower seeds, 1,
117–118
Sweet potatoes, 9

Tacitus, 113
Taurine, 127
Teeth, 47
Tel Aviv University, 47
Texas A&M University, 133
Dept. of Animal
Sciences, 64
Texas University, 133
Texturizers, 1
Theophrastus, 113
Thiamine. *See* Vitamin B_1.
Threonine, 94, 120, 123
Thymus gland, 123
Thyroid gland, 122
Thyroid hormones, 127
Tocopherols, 25
Tofu, 159
Tomatoes, 5, 14–16, 30, 62
juice, 62
Toxins, 19, 28–29, 141–142,
149
Triglycerides, 132
Trout, 1

Trypsin inhibitor, 157
Tryptophan, 123, 124
Tufts University, 63, 75, 76,
104, 130
Jean Mayer Human
Nutrition Research
Center on Aging, 40,
44, 45, 74, 96, 130
Turkeys, 139–140
stuffing, 140
Turmeric, 5
Tyrosine, 122, 127

Ultragrain White Whole
Wheat flour, 76
University of Arizona,
Tucson, 132, 133
University of California,
Davis, 6, 110
College of Agriculture
and Environmental
Sciences, 99
University of California,
San Francisco, 100
University of Florida
College of Medicine, 55
University of Georgia,
College of
Agricultural and
Environmental
Sciences, 108
University of Graz,
Austria, 39
University of Illinois,
Urbana–Champaign,
5, 137
University of Leeds, 87
University of Michigan,
52, 153
University of Minnesota,
67, 75
University of New Hamp-
shire Cooperative
Service, 46
University of Reading, 87

University of Scranton, 42
University of
Southampton, 49
University of Sydney, 84
University of Toronto, 15,
80, 98
University of Vermont, 146
University of Verona, Italy,
98
University of Western
Ontario, 56
Center for Human
Nutrition, 55
University of Wisconsin,
60
Food Research Institute,
152
Medical School
Coronary Thrombosis
Research Laboratory,
60
Urinary tract infections,
46–47
U.S. Department of
Agriculture, 4, 16, 32,
37, 43, 44, 45, 69, 72,
74, 77, 78, 84, 128, 136,
138, 150, 151
Agricultural Research
Service, 29, 40, 42, 56,
58, 61
Cooperative State
Research, Education,
and Extension Service,
33
Horticultural Research
Laboratory, 56
Meat and Poultry
Hotline, 139–140
U.S. Environmental
Protection Agency, 85
U.S. Food and Drug
Administration, 64, 76,
79, 88, 112, 141, 146,
158, 161

Utah State University, 143

Valine, 123
Vasodilators, 120
Vaughan, Beatrice, 33
Vegetables, 3–36
  bulb, 10–12
  buying and storing, 7
  canning, 32
  cruciferous, 8
  cucurbits, 9–10
  drying, 32–33
  freezing, 31–32
  "fruit," 12–16
  leafy green, 7–8
  other, 16
  preserving, 31–36
  raw vs cooked, 19–20,
    28–30
  retaining nutrients in
    cooked, 30
  root and tuberous, 8–9
  selecting, 16
  top-scoring for
    antioxidants, 6
  See also individual types.
Vegetarianism, 128–132,
  143–144
Very low-density
  lipoprotein (VLDL).
  See Cholesterol.
Victoria Hospital, Ontario,
  56
Vinegar, 24, 26–28
  apple-cider, 27
  balsamic, 26, 28
  beet, 28
  herb, 27
  homemade, 27–28
  malt, 27
  wine, 28

Vinson, Joe, 42
Vitamin A, 7, 13, 15, 18, 29,
  30, 48, 61, 152
Vitamin B complex, 13, 18,
  52, 68–69, 144
Vitamin B$_1$, 52, 61, 68
Vitamin B$_2$, 52, 68
Vitamin B$_3$, 18, 68, 123
Vitamin B$_6$, 61, 68, 131
Vitamin B$_{12}$, 131, 157
Vitamin C, 5, 7–8, 15, 16,
  18, 23, 29, 31, 32, 39,
  45, 48, 51, 52, 53,
  54–55, 61
Vitamin D, 30, 118, 134,
  152
Vitamin E, 5, 13, 24, 30, 39,
  45, 48, 51, 53, 60, 68,
  70, 103–104, 107, 108,
  118, 134, 152
Vitamin K, 30, 152, 158
Vitamins, 3

Wada, Leslie, 46
Walnuts, 1, 95, 97,
  100–101, 109–110
Watermelon, 1, 61–62
Watercress, 23
Wedzicha, Bronek L., 87
Weight, 73–75
Weiss, Ervin I., 47
Wheat, whole, 128
Wheat berry, whole, 1
Wheat bran, 2
Wheat germ, 2, 68
Whey, 82
WHO, 85–86, 88, 128, 129
Whole foods, 1–2, 3–36,
  37–66, 67–91, 93–118,
  119–161, 163–164
  defined, 1–2

Whole Grain Council, 78,
  79
Whole grains, 67–91
  acknowledging, 76–79
  blood pressure and, 72
  cancer and, 71
  defining, 78
  diabetes and, 73
  glycemic index and,
    83–85
  heart disease and,
    71–72
  learning and, 75–76
  longevity and, 75
  obesity and, 73–75
  preparing, 82–83
  recovering, 69–70
  sensitivity to, 88–91
  shopping for, 70–82
  strokes and, 72–73
Williams, Roger J., 136
Wine, red, 59
Wirthlin Worldwide, 53
Wolf, Ray, 33
Wolfe, Bernard M., 131
Women's Health Study, 75
World Health
  Organization. See
  WHO.
World War II, 44, 77, 113,
  148

Yersinia enterocolitica, 64
Yogurt, 1, 144–145
Yogurt cheese, making,
  147
Yonsei University, Korea,
  71

Zinc, 68–69
Zucchini, 9–10

About the Author

Beatrice Trum Hunter has written numerous books on food issues, including *Consumer Beware: Your Food & What's Been Done to It* (Simon & Schuster, 1971), *The Mirage of Safety: Food Additives & Federal Policy* (Charles Scribners' Sons, 1975), *The Great Nutrition Robbery* (Charles Scribners' Sons, 1978), *The Sugar Trap & How to Avoid It* (Houghton Mifflin, 1982), and *Food & Your Health* (Basic Health Publications, 2003). As food editor for more than twenty years at *Consumers' Research Magazine,* her monthly columns and feature articles brought cutting-edge issues before general recognition.

Hunter has received many awards and recognitions for her work. The International Academy of Preventive Medicine made her an honorary fellow. Other honorary memberships include the American Academy of Environmental Medicine, the Price-Pottenger Nutrition Foundation, the Weston A. Price Foundation, and Nutrition for Optimal Health. She received the prestigious Jonathan Forman Award, was honored by the International College of Applied Nutrition, and was recipient of the President's Award by the National Nutritional Foods Association.